T0133419

Managing Obesity in the Workplace

Managing Obesity in the Workplace

NERYS WILLIAMS

Consultant Occupational Physician, Birmingham
Former Honorary Consultant in Weight Management,
Heart of England NHS Trust, Birmingham

Foreword by

SUDHESH KUMAR

Professor of Medicine, Diabetes and Metabolism
Warwick Medical School

Radcliffe Publishing
Oxford • New York

Radcliffe Publishing Ltd
18 Marcham Road
Abingdon
Oxon OX14 1AA
United Kingdom

www.radcliffe-oxford.com

Electronic catalogue and worldwide online ordering facility.

British Library Cataloguing in Publication Data

A catalogue record for this book is available from the British Library.

ISBN-13: 978 1 84619 058 2

Typeset by Pindar New Zealand (Egan Reid), Auckland, New Zealand
Printed in the United Kingdom by Hobbs the Printers Ltd, Totton, Hampshire

Contents

Foreword   vii

Preface   ix

About the author   xi

1 Introduction: an overview   1

2 The background and scale of the obesity problem   7

3 The medical consequences of obesity   15

4 The workplace implications of obesity: the fit between worker
   and workplace   23

5 Prejudice and discrimination in employment and healthcare   31

6 Current management of obesity   41

7 The workplace setting: improving nutrition and promoting
   physical activity   53

8 Workplace design: improving nutrition and promoting physical
   activity   69

9A Health promotion: work task and workplace redesign and
    population approaches   75

9B Health promotion: the individual approach   83

10 Legal aspects of obesity and the *Disability Discrimination Act*   93

11 Further resources   99

Appendix 1:   Common questions and answers   105

Appendix 2:   Food labelling   107

Appendix 3:   Popular diets, past and present   109

Appendix 4:   Suggested eight-week programme for weight loss
               in a workplace   113

Appendix 5:   Suggested healthy substitutions for traditional
               workplace buffet lunches   117

Appendix 6:   Examples of nutritional interventions and increased
               physical activity   119

Appendix 7:   American College of Occupational and Environmental
               Medicine 2004 Labor Day checklist on obesity   123

Index   127

Foreword

Managing Obesity in the Workplace is the result of the author's perception of a need for a book that synthesises current knowledge on issues relating to obesity in the workplace and its management. We are all acutely aware of the epidemic of overweight and obesity across the world. Clearly, changes in eating habits and the ready availability of energy-dense foods are major contributors, as is significant reduction in physical activity during leisure time and at work. We spend about a third of our lives at work and the world of work has changed very dramatically in the last 20 years. Most jobs have now become obesogenic – we have systematically reduced physical activity from them to improve efficiency and productivity. Yet, during this time we have paid relatively little attention to the role that the workplace plays in creating obesity. Furthermore, some of the policies currently adopted in the workplace may aggravate obesity in susceptible individuals and there is often little support for people who wish to lose weight and little help to prevent them gaining weight at work.

What can be done? First, the workplace can be made less obesogenic if some thought is given to schemes to provide for physical activity and also to ensure that the environment is safe for obese individuals to continue to contribute to the work of the organisation. Changing the environment in this way may involve looking at food choices available and also making it possible to incorporate physical activity. Some action to improve the 'fit' between the worker and the workplace may help obese individuals to continue to work and be productive in a safe environment. Finally, in some instances, offering weight management solutions at the workplace may also be appropriate.

It is encouraging to see that such a book has been produced at all and it couldn't be more timely. Most indices for obesity are still heading in the wrong direction, however there are a number of significant strides being made in reducing obesity and its related complications. This book provides practical examples, ideas and case studies suitable for all types and sizes of businesses and is, I believe, a 'one-stop shop' for all issues around obesity and the workplace that are facing employers and staff today. Reducing levels of obesity may seem a distant goal now, but it is one worth striving for. This book will be valuable to those who wish to contribute to this goal by changing the workplace and making it a healthier environment.

Professor Sudhesh Kumar
University of Warwick
August 2007

Preface

The epidemic of obesity is now affecting all continents and most countries of the world. It has not happened overnight but changes to lifestyle have led to steady weight gain of increasing numbers of people and this is having a profound effect on their health. Obesity is expensive, both in personal and societal terms, and every angle needs to be explored to help people manage their weight better and prevent weight gain.

My interest in obesity and work arose from clinical work in the National Health Service, where I saw patient after patient struggling with their weight and with their job – if they had one. Unemployment was high in our population of clinic attendees and so was reliance on disability benefits. The patients often said that they had little sympathy offered to them and no support and that they often felt discriminated against. It became clear though that the interaction between obesity and work was far wider, and the more I read around the topic, the more I realised that there were real health and safety issues from conditions occurring with obesity, such as sleep apnoea (particularly in drivers), and in the ability of people who were obese to use protective equipment properly.

I also found that relatively little attention had been paid to these impacts of obesity on the world of work. Looking in the health and safety, ergonomics and attendance management literature, I found that obesity did not even get a mention.

This book aims to fill some of the gaps and to provide its readers with an overview of the issues across occupational health and also to provide suggestions of what can be achieved in their workplaces by using case studies from around the world.

The workplace offers a different venue to pass on key messages and provide information to populations. These populations are, to a certain degree, 'captive' and the fact that so many people are often together in one place, means that interventions can be efficient as well as effective. But we must not forget that the majority of businesses in every country are small- and medium-sized enterprises, so the book includes some examples of what can be achieved using few resources other than enthusiasm.

Such is the speed of the spread of obesity that we must investigate every avenue, not just the healthcare system, in order to encourage people to eat sensibly and to take physical activity. The workplace could be designed to facilitate this but all too often work is organised to be 'obesogenic' and the work environment encourages rather than dissuades excess calorie consumption.

I hope that by showing obesity's consequences, at a population level but also at the individual level, and its impact on so many areas of business, I will encourage workplace-based action. I hope I have provided the ammunition that readers need to convince opinion leaders in their workplaces to devote resources to this crucial issue.

The book is aimed at occupational health doctors and nurses but also health promotion specialists who perhaps are not as familiar with wider occupational workplace issues. But I hope it will also be of interest to other occupational health and safety professionals, such as safety officers and ergonomists, managers and worker representatives as well – the more people who realise what needs to be done, the more likely it is that things will happen. And happen they must, if we are to successfully address the epidemic, prevent the health decline and have a workforce capable of the many economic challenges ahead.

Nerys Williams
August 2007

About the author

Nerys Williams qualified in Medicine from Manchester University and then undertook a series of hospital posts before completing her training and accreditation in General Practice. She then joined the Wellcome Foundation Limited to undertake specialist training in Occupational Medicine, which was completed in 1992.

From 1992 to 2004 she worked for the Health and Safety Executive, latterly as a Senior Medical Inspector and Head of the Employment Medical Advisory Service.

She now works as Principal Occupational Physician for the UK Department for Work and Pensions but also worked as Honorary Consultant in Obesity Medicine/ Weight Management in Heartlands and Solihull NHS Trust up to 2005.

Her current occupational interests centre around obesity, and disability and rehabilitation, and workplace modifications to improve health.

She is a Fellow of the Royal College of Physicians of London, a Fellow of the Faculty of Occupational Medicine (London) and is the author of two other occupational health books and over 50 peer-reviewed papers.

I would like to thank my close friends and family for their continuous encouragement and support.

CHAPTER 1

Introduction: an overview

'The situation has reached crisis point and
current policies are failing.'

TRUST FOR AMERICA'S HEALTH, AUGUST 2005

THE BIGGER PICTURE FOR BUSINESS

According to the World Health Organization (WHO), we are in the grip of an obesity epidemic.[1] Put simply, this means that more than 15% of the people in this country, the UK, are suffering from the condition. But obesity is not just a UK issue – it is a worldwide phenomenon which has significant implications both for public health and for business.

Such is the impact of obesity at the individual level that it has been described as 'the main preventable cause of illness and premature death in the US', overtaking smoking, for the first time, in 2005.[2]

Obesity is an important condition, which deserves our attention as workplace health advisors and the attention of business for several reasons.

- It is a very common condition, affecting over one in five adults in the UK and US at present.
- It is predicted to become even more prevalent over the next decade.
- It is associated with a large number of other medical conditions, co-morbidities, which cause pain, suffering, reduced productivity and absence from work.
- Obesity is life limiting – an obese person at the age of 40 years can expect to die seven years earlier than someone of normal weight.[3]
- The size, weight and personal dimensions of obese workers have implications

1

for the fit of personal protective equipment and uniforms. Custom-made clothing and masks can lead to increased costs, as can custom-made chairs and workstations. Air travel may be prohibitively expensive if two seats need to be booked for an obese traveller.

∎ Because of the prejudice and discrimination shown towards obese people from healthcare providers, HR and personnel professionals and line mangers, businesses may at best lose out on real talent and, at worst, contravene disability discrimination legislation.

∎ Overweight and obesity are now so common that businesses have to remain aware that the way they treat their staff may also have an impact on the perception of the business by their customers, many of whom will also be overweight and obese. Recently the media had a feeding frenzy when the human resources director of a health club reportedly circulated a memo on the negative aspects on its staff of 'larger employees'. Such 'own goals' in an industry which targets weight reduction can harm business viability.

∎ The changing demographics of the Western world mean that there will be older workers in the workforce in future. This is already occurring due to financial and social pressures. Obesity rises with age, so it is likely that the number of obese and overweight workers will also increase.

CHANGING DEMOGRAPHICS

We live in a fast-moving global village with significant demographic changes already affecting the supply of labour and the type of labour.

Rising rates of overweight and obese workers are occurring against a background of:

∎ fewer entrants to the labour market due to:
  ∎ falling birth rates since the 1980s
  ∎ workers entering the labour market later, due to longer time spent in education (more people with degrees)
  ∎ increased numbers of people claiming health conditions and incapacity from work and so not being available for work[4]
  ∎ increased numbers of obese children – our future workers. Some businesses are already finding that young new entrants are unfit and unable to carry out physical jobs in manufacturing. The years of physical inactivity have taken their toll and produced new entrants to the world of work who are unhealthier than people 40 years older than themselves.

But there are also greater numbers of people leaving the labour market due to:

∎ expectations of early retirement
∎ ill-health retirement
∎ the natural retirement of the 'baby boomer' generation.

Employers may find it difficult to find their 'usual' type of worker. They will need older workers and those who have chronic health conditions, as labour may become in short supply.

CASE STUDY 1.1

A call centre in the West Midlands had difficulty attracting and retaining staff, so it set about exploring ways of competing with other businesses to attract skilled operators. The company identified a workplace champion who sought the views of workers and produced a report to the management. The report identified that improvements to the working environment – in terms of décor of the centre, flexibility of working teams and better access to healthy food – were all valued by staff.

The management addressed the issues and, in the case of better nutrition, they refurbished the tea points, installed microwave ovens to allow food to be brought in from home and provided water fountains on each floor. They also liaised with local sandwich vendors and ensured that a range of healthy options, including fruit, were available and negotiated a discount with a local organic fruit and vegetable delivery service. They felt the exercise had improved working relationships in the business.

Businesses thus need to attract and retain talented workers, as competition has never been greater with economies such as those of Russia and China increasing their output of trade at a phenomenal rate. China is reported to be doubling exports every two years, with labour costs of only 5% of those of the European Union (EU),[5] and countries such as India are leading the way with highly skilled technology graduates. More competition for Western business means more attention is needed to the costs and bottom line.

Against this background of economic activity, EU countries have to compete with their increasingly older workforces, reduced labour supply and increased burden of chronic ill-health, due to conditions such as obesity, in those who are at work.

The UK National Audit Office has estimated the economic impact of obesity; the estimate for 1998 is as follows.

Obesity costs for England alone:
- £0.5 billion in NHS treatment for obesity directly and its associated diseases
- £2 billion in indirect costs
- 18 million sick days
- 40 000 lost years of working life.

NAO Report: Tackling Obesity in England, February 2001. (Reproduced with permission from the NAO. Copyright NAO.)

But the issue is one not just for business but also for Governments as well, as the number of people working compared to those who are dependent (i.e. the young and the elderly) is rising, putting stress on the social and healthcare support network.

The country needs (and that means we, too, need):
▌ more people working
▌ more healthy workers
▌ more productive workers
▌ more people working for longer.

And the numbers required will not be delivered just by an expanding EU and migration of people. So, in order to achieve these aims, we need to address the reasons why people work for less time and less effectively and efficiently, and that means addressing common modifiable risk factors for chronic ill-health, the prime one being obesity.

Government has only recently really become aware to the health impacts of obesity. In the White Paper, *Choosing Health: making healthy choices easier*, published in 2004,[6] the Government outlined its intentions towards obesity. It has set a number of aims and initiatives, including:
▌ commissioning work by the National Institute for Clinical Excellence (NICE) to produce definitive guidance on the prevention, identification, management and treatment of obesity (now published)
▌ developing a 'care pathway' for obesity patients, raising awareness, providing information, advice and referral to specialist services
▌ producing a Government-commissioned weight loss guide to help people choose the best regimen for them to lose weight
▌ commissioning research where there are gaps in the evidence of what works
▌ supporting the setting-up of an obesity partnership body
▌ producing a 'patient activity questionnaire' to help assess the needed for exercise referral.

But none of these initiatives relates to the workplace, which is briefly mentioned as a possible site for health promotion, and there is no recognition of the impact of obesity on employment and working life.

Many actions still fall far short of being able to have a dramatic effect on the prevalence of the condition.

Across Whitehall, the seat of the UK Government, departments are committed to addressing physical activity and better nutrition – *see* Figure 1.1 – but the message seems to be directed largely for the benefit of children. Whilst this is important – indeed, as it involves our future workers, its emphasis is not unreasonable on economic grounds – the lack of any tangible initiatives and investment for adults is disappointing. The key message for business is that it should not wait for any Government initiatives but rather should grasp the problem to ensure its own profitability and sustainability.

Occupational health and safety practitioners, health promotion specialists and public health professionals are all key to raising awareness of the need for such action, but it is business – and particularly business which relies heavily on human capital – that will be the key initiator, driver and beneficiary of such action in the workplace.

Providing a healthy workplace with opportunities for a healthy lifestyle will help business to meet the challenge of changes in labour supply and competition. To do this we need to:

▮ provide information and support
▮ alter some work tasks
▮ modify the work environment
▮ provide increased opportunities for increased physical activity and better nutrition.

This does not always need to mean increased expense but rather doing things differently and considering how to develop a healthy workforce and workplace when designing work and the work environment.

▮ Develop a broader strategy to combat obesity in the whole population.
(Responsible departments: Department of Health, Department for Education and Skills, Department for Culture, Media and Sport)

▮ Increase the uptake of sporting and cultural opportunities by young people and adults.
(Responsible department: Department for Culture, Media and Sport)

▮ Enhance access to culture and sport for children, including increasing the percentage of school children spending a minimum of two hours per week on PE and school sport from 25% to 85% by 2008.
(Responsible department: Department for Education and Skills, Department for Culture, Media and Sport)

▮ Improve the quality and sustainability of local environments and neighbourhoods with more clean, safe green spaces and a better quality of built environment.
(Responsible department: Office of the Deputy Prime Minister)

FIGURE 1.1 Aims and targets of Government departments.

KEY POINTS

∞   Obesity is a key issue for business sustainability.

∞   It is likely to become more important as the population ages and demographic changes occur.

∞   Addressing obesity in the workplace need not be expensive or complex.

∞   Doing nothing is unlikely to be an option – the only choice for companies is to deal with the condition or its complications, including other medical conditions, sickness absence, disability and early retirements due to poor health.

REFERENCES

1 WHO. *Obesity: preventing and managing the global epidemic*. Geneva: WHO; 1998.

2 Mokdad AH, Marks JS, Stroup DF *et al*. Actual causes of death in the United States 2000. *JAMA*. 2005; **291**: 1238–45. (Erratum *JAMA*. 2005; **293**: 293–94.)

3 Peeters A, Barendregt JJ, Willekens F *et al*. NEDCOM, the Netherlands Epidemiology and Demography Compression of Morbidity Research Group. Obesity in adulthood and its consequences for life expectancy: a life table analysis. *Ann Intern Med*. 2003; **138**: 24–32.

4 www.dwp.gov.uk (accessed 29 December 2005).

5 Speech by Lord Philip Hunt, UK Minister Department for Work and Pensions, at a conference in Cardiff, 2005.

6 Department of Health. *Choosing Health: making healthy choices easier*. 2004 www.dh.gov.uk (accessed March 2006).

CHAPTER 2

The background and scale of the obesity problem

'Genes load the gun but environment pulls the trigger.'

GEORGE BRAY, 1996

In order to successfully prevent and manage obesity in the workplace, it is necessary to be clear about some basic definitions used in obesity and understand their limitations and why they are important. It is also useful to understand why we have such increasing rates of obesity and the role of genes and environment in causation.

WHAT IS OBESITY AND HOW CAN IT BE MEASURED?

Obesity has been defined by the Royal College of Physicians in the UK as 'a disorder in which excess fat has accumulated to an extent that health maybe adversely affected'.[1] Usually people are obese when their body mass index (BMI) exceeds a fixed level, but weight is the most popular measure of body fat and, for many individuals, including employees, weight is the most important factor. It has the advantage that its calculation is cheap, quick and easily understood. It is also the most common yardstick by which success at weight reduction is measured. However, it is crude and can be misleading, as it takes no account of height or of the relative contribution of bone and muscle to weight.

For this reason, the definition of obesity is based on the *body mass index (BMI)*. BMI is calculated by measuring weight and height (in clothing but without shoes) and then performing the following calculation:

$$BMI = weight/height^2$$

BMI is used as a surrogate for body fat and has been used in the large-scale studies which look at the increased risks from being overweight and obese.

But as a measure it can be misleading, as very muscular individuals such as elite athletes and active sportspeople who run marathons or triathlons or frequently row or cycle may have a raised BMI. This is because muscle weighs more than fat, and so very muscular individuals can have high BMIs but low body fat levels. They are not at increased risk of the many health complications of a person with a high BMI due to high body fat.

Standard BMI charts are available and are useful for estimation of fat in adults, but specialised charts are needed for adolescents and children in whom growth spurts influence ranges.

The World Health Organization (WHO) has determined that a normal BMI is $18.5–24.9 \text{ kg/m}^2$, overweight is 25–29.9 and obesity $> 30 \text{ kg/m}^2$.

TABLE 2.1 WHO definition of overweight and obesity

Classification	BMI (kg/m²)	Risk of co-morbidities
Normal range	18.5–24.9	average
Overweight	25.0–29.9	increased
Obese class I	30.0–34.9	moderate
Obese class II	35.0–39.9	severe
Obese class III	> 40.0	very severe

But these arbitrary cut-offs relate to Caucasian populations. Because of the increased risk of cardiovascular disease in populations from South Asia, the values for this group have been set lower.

In Asian populations, a BMI $> 23 \text{ kg/m}^2$ should be considered as overweight and a BMI $> 25 \text{ kg/m}^2$ is obese.[2] This has implications for any standard setting in working populations.

TABLE 2.2 Table of body mass index for different ethnic groups (kg/m²)

	Caucasian	South Asian
Overweight	> 25	> 23
Obese	> 30	> 25

But BMI is not the only indirect estimate of body fat. All fat is not equal in its ability to lead to ill-health and chronic disease. The fat that lies around the abdomen (producing the pear-shaped body), as opposed to the fat which collects around the thighs (producing the apple-shaped body), is more metabolically active and produces a host of hormones and active chemicals which affect risks to health. This so-called *truncal (abdominal) obesity* is associated with the presence of other risk factors for heart disease, including insulin resistance, decreased

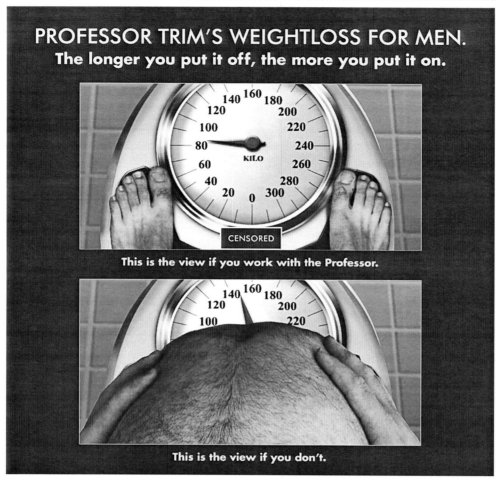

PROFESSOR TRIM'S WEIGHTLOSS FOR MEN.
The longer you put it off, the more you put it on.

This is the view if you work with the Professor.

This is the view if you don't.

Professor Trims, from the developers of GutBusters. The world's first scientifically designed weight loss program for men.

If you're an Australian man, you can expect to put on an average of 8kg from age 30 to 50[1]. And that's just the average! In fact, nearly 70% of over 35 year olds are overweight or obese, and 1 in 3 has diabetes or pre-diabetes as a result[2].

Of course, this doesn't apply to you. And anyway, you can always lose it when you want. Can't you?

So why is it getting harder to see where it's getting softer?

Try this: Measure around your waist at the navel with a standard tape measure. If you're more than 102cm (more than 90cm for Indians and Asians), you're in line for failing eyesight, impotency and a range of other health problems[3]. You could benefit from making friends with the Professor – like over 100,000 other Aussie men have since 1990.

Professor Trims is Australia's only men's 'waist removalist' program. Developed by the makers of GutBusters, with 10 of the world's leading obesity professors, the Professor Trim program approaches weight loss in 3 stages – 3 weeks, 3 months, and for life – to make sure that you not only get rid of that spare 'lunch', but keep it off.

With resources that range from meal replacements, to personal support, to information packs including audio and video CDs and meal plans, Professor Trims uses the latest scientific knowledge in an at-home, group or medical environment - without the gimmicks.

Says Ted Anderson, who lost the 12kg he couldn't shake since Vietnam:

❝ My wife laughed when I said I was going on another weight loss program. We're both laughing – and dancing and enjoying things - a whole lot more now. ❞

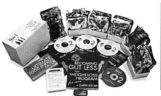

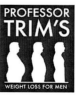

Call 1800 100 550, visit www.professortrim.com or ask your pharmacist*.

1. Australian Institute of Health and Welfare, 2003 figures 2. AusDiab study, 2002 3. World Health Organisation, 2002. * see web-site for details

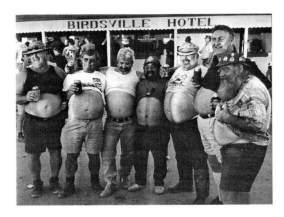

glucose tolerance, decreased HDL cholesterol, elevated LDL cholesterol and triglycerides and hypertension – known as metabolic syndrome. Depositing fat around the abdomen leads to an increase in the circumference of the waist and a reduction in the waist:hip ratio, and it is these two measurements which are increasingly used in studies and programmes to measure the benefits of weight loss in terms of reduction of risks to health.

As with BMI, there are ethnic differences in cut-off points, as shown in Table 2.3, but unusually there are also differences accepted by different groups such as Europeans (Europids)[2] and Americans, Japanese, Chinese and other ethnic groups, which are derived from different criteria and estimates.[3]

TABLE 2.3 Waist circumferences for men and women (WHO)[2]

	Europids[2]	Americans[3]	South Asians[2]
Men	< 102 cms	< 94 cms	< 90 cms
Women	< 88 cms	< 80 cms	< 80 cms

However, the risk of obesity-associated metabolic complications increases *above 94 cms for European men and 80 cms for European women*, therefore these measurements would be more appropriate to use in the workplace setting to encourage weight (and particularly abdominal fat) loss.

Body fat estimations

It is also possible to estimate total body fat using either skin fold calipers or electronic methods. Using skin fold callipers requires training and there is large inter-measurement variability. Electronic impedance methods are now more generally established and use either a set of scales, measuring impedance via the feet, or can be hand held. Measuring body fat along with weight, BMI and waist circumference can help in identifying success in weight reduction programmes and in motivating employees.

THE SCALE OF THE PROBLEM

Having established the commonly used definitions of obesity, it is now important to look at the scale of the problem facing healthcare professionals, employers and employees.

It is not just the number of people who are overweight and obese which is the important issue, but also the rate of increase in their numbers. This is happening virtually all over the world and particularly in developing countries such as China.

The current prevalence (number of cases) of obesity in industrialised countries is between 14% and 20%.[2] The US has for many years led the way in the number of obese and overweight people, but the UK has the fastest growth rate of overweight and obese children in the world.

In the US, headline figures include:

▮ in 2004, the adult obesity rate rose in 48 states and nationally from 23.7% to 24.5%[5]
▮ in 10 US states, over 25% of adults are now obese[5]
▮ the states with the highest percentage of obese inhabitants are Mississippi (29.5%), followed by Alabama (28.9%) and West Virginia (27.6%) (Centers for Disease Control and Prevention)[5]
▮ currently 64.5% of US adults are either overweight or obese
▮ according to projections, 73% will be overweight or obese by 2008.

The picture in the UK is equally disturbing. The Health Survey for England and Wales revealed a nearly three-fold increase in cases of obesity in men and nearly four-fold in women over a 20-year period (*see* Table 2.4).[4]

TABLE 2.4 Results of the Health Survey for England and Wales[4]: percentage of people obese

	1980	1990	2000
Men	8%	12%	> 21%
Women	6%	8%	> 21%

Projections for the UK suggest that by 2010, over 25% of people will be obese. More detailed information on projected rates in the future can be found in a recently published forecasting document, *Forecasting obesity to 2010*, 25 August 2006, which can be downloaded free of charge from www.dh.gov.uk/publications andstatistics

CAUSES OF OBESITY

There has been a long debate about the role of genetics versus the environment in determining weight gain and weight loss and the causes of the epidemic of obesity currently affecting the Western world. On the genetic side of the argument, there are a few rare gene mutations which lead to gross obesity which presents in childhood. Similar gene mutations occur in mice and other rodents. But these are extremely rare and account for only a handful of very obese children in the country.

We know more about the role of genes and our genetic make-up from studies which have been undertaken on adopted twins. Studies of adopted children show that the weight of the biological mother and, to a lesser extent, the biological father, are greater predictors of weight in the child than the weights of their adoptive parents, suggesting a stronger genetic component than an environmental one.[6] Overfeeding studies in twins also suggest that genetic factors influence who gains weight and how much they gain.[7] Overall, twin studies suggest that about 50% or more of the variation between individuals in BMI has a genetic basis.[8]

However, the gene pool cannot have changed significantly in the last 20 years to explain the huge rise in the numbers of people who are overweight or obese. So environmental factors are likely to be highly significant. We know that our lifestyle has changed considerably over the last 20–30 years and it is no coincidence that the adult phase of weight gain in men corresponds with the fall in time spent on leisure sports. There have been major changes since the 1960s in increased car ownership, labour-saving domestic appliances, use of television and computers and a reduction in jobs requiring physical activity. In short, people expend much less energy on their daily activities than they used to and, coupled with age-related changes in metabolism, they gain weight as they age, up to about 70 years of age.

Changes in physical activity have occurred at the same time as changes in eating patterns and types of food consumed. Social commentators who observed the needs of men undertaking physically active jobs found that they consumed 3000–4000 calories per day in 3–4 main meals. As lifestyles changed, meals became fewer, breakfast was often omitted and lunch was no longer a hot meal. Now some people have no breakfast but continually snack all day on energy-dense food which overrides the body's natural mechanisms of food intake regulation. Sugar-rich foods also bypass appetite regulation and the combination of fat and sugary foods activate pleasure centres in the brain – so no surprise if people seek them out. It is also known that the visual impact of larger portions reduces appetite regulation in both adults and children – so no wonder large portion sizes are promoted for home and restaurant consumption.

'Meal deals' which encourage increased consumption of calories and 'super-sizing' – the payment of a small amount of extra money for a large increase in portion – have become attractive as they encourage eating 'on the move'. Sitting down and just eating concentrates the mind and appetite regulation on food consumption. Distraction techniques such as encouraging eating while walking along the street or at a company buffet lunch mean that large numbers of calories can be consumed without appetite regulation kicking in or any comprehension of the true number of calories ingested. Depending on the type of food, if it is high in fat and low in protein, it may not even be satisfying and so, despite thousands of calories being taken in, the person becomes hungry and eats again.

Other causes of and predisposing factors for obesity are shown in Box 2.1, but it should be remembered that endocrine or glandular problems are rare. Far more common are drugs and medicines prescribed for a wide range of conditions. These are shown in Box 2.2.

It is really no surprise that we have such high rates of obesity. After all, the situation can be summarised as 'nature loads the gun and the environment pulls the trigger'.

BOX 2.1 Predisposing factors for obesity and causes of obesity

Predisposing factors for obesity
- Age (obesity increases with age)
- Gender (women are more likely to gain weight than men)
- Social class (unskilled workers are more likely than professionals to be obese)
- Genes/heredity (*see* text)
- Marital status (married people are more likely to be obese than singles)

Causes of obesity
- Reduced physical activity
- Calorie intake imbalance compared to need
- Smoking cessation
- Disorders of the sympatho-adrenal system
- Rarely endocrine disorders such as hypothyroidism
- Drugs/medication (*see* Box 2.2).

BOX 2.2 Common 'obesogenic' drugs

- Antipsychotics
- Antidepressants (including tricyclics, selective serotonin-reuptake inhibitors, monoamine oxidase inhibitors, lithium)
- Anticonvulsants (phenytoin, sodium valproate)
- Corticosteroids
- Oral contraceptives and drugs containing progestagens
- Insulin
- Oral hypoglycaemic agents
- Older antihistamines.

KEY POINTS

∞   Obesity is caused by both environmental and genetic factors.

∞   By 2010 it is predicted that more than 25% of the UK population will be obese.

∞   Obesity is a worldwide health problem.

REFERENCES

1 *Storing Up Problems: the medical case for a slimmer nation.* Report of working party. London: Royal College of Physicians; 2003.

2 WHO. Obesity: preventing and managing the global epidemic. WHO Technical Report Series number 894. Geneva: WHO; 2000.

3 James WPDT. Assessing obesity: are ethnic differences in body mass and waist circumference justified? *Obes Rev* 2005; **6**: 179–81.

4 Joint Health Surveys Unit (on behalf of the Department of Health). *Health Survey for England 2002.* London: The Stationery Office; 2003.

5 US people getting fatter, fast. www.news.bbc.co.uk/1/hi/health/4183086.stm (accessed 25 August 2005).

6 Stunkard AJ, Sorensen TI, Hanis C *et al.* An adoption study of human obesity. *NEJM* 1986; **314** (4); 193.

7 Bouchard C, Tremblay A, Depres JP *et al.* The response to long term feeding in identical twins. *NEJM* 1990; **322**: 1477–82.

8 Allison DB, Matz PE, Pietrobelli A *et al.* Genetic and environmental influences on obesity. In: Bendich A, Deckelbaum RJ, editors. *Primary and Secondary Preventive Nutrition.* Totowa, NJ: Humana Press; 2001: 147–64.

CHAPTER 3

The medical consequences of obesity

'Corpulence is not only a disease itself. It is a
harbinger of others.'

HIPPOCRATES

Obesity is now recognised as a chronic disease which has a significant impact on physical and psychological health and on social interaction.

The medical complications of the condition affect almost every system in the body, with most studies relying on either body mass index or, more rarely, waist circumference or waist:hip ratio to define the population and determine the risks.

MORTALITY

The graph of body mass index and mortality is U or J shaped. Put simply, under-weight and obese people have increased risk of mortality when compared to people of 'normal weight'. The association between low BMI and higher mortality is in part due to cigarette smoking, but the association at all BMIs weakens as people age.

DIABETES

Obesity is the main driver behind the rising rates of diabetes seen in the UK. Whereas in the so-called type 1 diabetes, there is a complete lack of insulin production, in the type 2 diabetes, seen in association with obesity, it is insulin resistance which is the main problem. The link between obesity and diabetes is strong both within and between ethnic groups, with over 75% of diabetics being either overweight or obese.

The risk of developing diabetes does not just begin when a person becomes overweight or obese – risks increase from BMIs as low as 22 kg/m² in women and 24 kg/m² in men and this risk increases at even lower rates (an estimated 1–2 kg/m² less) in Asian populations. There is a 25% increase in relative risk for developing diabetes with every 1 kg/m² increase in BMI above 22 kg/m² and the risk increases as BMI increases.

Women with a BMI > 25 kg/m² have a 5-fold increased risk.
But women with a BMI >35 kg/m² have a 93-fold increased risk.
And in men with a BMI > 35 kg/m² there is a 42-fold increased risk[2,3]

Abdominal fat distribution, as measured by waist circumference, is also an independent risk factor for type 2 diabetes. This deposition of fat in the abdomen is associated with insulin resistance, which occurs in the tissues and in the liver.

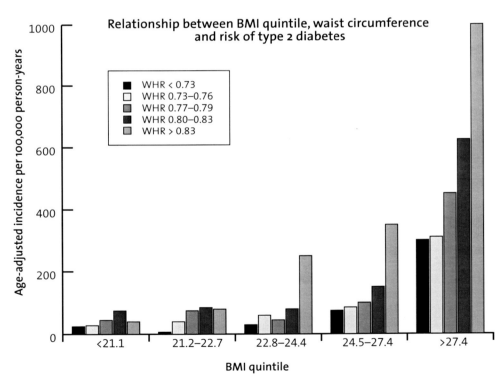

FIGURE 3.1 Age-adjusted incidence rates of non-insulin-dependent diabetes mellitus per 100 000 person-years (standardised to the age distribution of the Nurses' Health Study cohort), cross-classified according to the quintile of body mass index (BMI) and waist hip ratio (WHR). Reproduced with permission of *American Journal of Epidemiology*.

Initially the body can cope and produces more insulin to try to compensate but gradually the pancreas becomes 'burnt out' and so frank diabetes develops.

A constellation of symptoms such as insulin resistance, hypertension and altered cholesterol levels is known as the 'metabolic syndrome'.

CARDIOVASCULAR DISEASE

The most common and serious effects of obesity are seen on the heart and blood vessels. Obesity is associated with increased risk of heart attacks, hypertension and strokes. In an obese person, the heart has to work harder to pump blood to meet the increased demands of a greater body mass, thus *congestive heart failure* is an important cause of death.

Hypertension is seen in more than a third of obese adults, who have twice the rate of high blood pressure when compared to those with a BMI of less than 25 kg/m². It has been estimated that for every 10% increase in weight, there is a 6 mmHg increase in systolic blood pressure and a 4 mm increase in diastolic blood pressure.

Coronary heart disease (CHD) also increases as obesity increases. The Nurses Health Study has shown that, after controlling for common confounders (such as smoking, age, etc.), the risk of CHD doubles between BMIs of 22–23 kg/m² and 25–28.9 kg/m² and is more than triple above 30 kg/m² compared to BMI of 21 kg/m².

RESPIRATORY PROBLEMS

Obesity also causes impaired respiratory function, particularly on lying flat, and can later lead to pulmonary hypertension and right-sided heart failure. One particularly important respiratory condition, which is seen in obese people, is known as *sleep apnoea*. Clinically presenting with very loud snoring and episodes when breathing stops altogether for 10–15 seconds at a time, it is caused by the deposition of fat in the neck and around the trachea. This reduces the diameter of the upper airway and, combined with increased fat in the abdominal cavity, which also reduces the lung volume, the problem is accentuated. The lack of breathing, reduced lung volume and narrowed airway result in reduced oxygen entering the lungs and therefore the blood and brain. When this reaches a critical point, this hypoxaemia causes the person to abruptly wake up. The condition is important as it leads to daytime sleepiness, irritability and aggressiveness with short-term memory loss and impaired concentration. The repeated episodes of hypoxaemia can also result in pulmonary hypertension.

People with sleep apnoea are not only less productive and may fall asleep at their desks during the day, but they have been reported to be at increased risk of both occupational[4] and road traffic accidents.[5] In addition to the classic history of excessively loud snoring and stopping breathing during sleep, a neck circumference of greater than 42 cm in men and greater than 40.5 cm in women can also predict sleep apnoea. The condition is effectively treated with continuous positive pressure (CPAP) applied via a facemask and worn at night at home.

CANCERS

Obesity has been reported to be one of the most important preventable causes of cancer. It has been estimated that about 10% of all non-smoking-related cancers are due to obesity, with being overweight and physically inactive accounting for 25–33% of cancers of the:

- breast
- colon
- uterus
- kidney
- oesophagus.[6]

And obesity has been linked to increased:

- asthma (in children)
- polycystic ovary syndrome (leading to infertility, hirsutism and menstrual irregularity. It has been estimated that obesity accounts for about 6% of all primary infertility)
- menorrhagia/heavy periods
- fatty liver
- gallstones (although the association is strongest for women and in people with BMIs > 45 kg/m^2)
- kidney disease
- gout
- varicose veins
- osteoarthritis.

The relative risks for the above conditions and others have been outlined by the National Audit Office and are shown in Box 3.1.

Most recently studies have also shown an increased risk of dementia and Alzheimers disease in people who have a raised body mass index in mid-life.[7]

BOX 3.1 Relative risk of health problems associated with obesity

Disease	Women	Men
Type 2 diabetes	12.7	5.2
Hypertension	4.2	2.6
Myocardial infarction	3.2	1.5
Colon cancer	2.7	3.0
Angina	1.8	1.8
Gall bladder disease	1.8	1.8
Ovarian cancer	1.7	–
Osteoarthritis	1.4	1.9
Stroke	1.3	1.3

NAO Report: Tackling Obesity in England, February 2001 (reproduced with permission of the NAO. Copyright NAO.)

PSYCHOLOGICAL CONSEQUENCES

Obesity has not only medical but also psychological features. Studies performed in the community and in patients attending obesity clinics differ in their results as far as depression and other mental health problems are concerned. Attendees at hospital and healthcare clinics have higher rates of depression than those in the community, but this may suggest a biased population seeking treatment. Low mood and loss of self-esteem are common in obese patients, as is the use of food both as a punishment and as a reward. Discrimination and prejudice towards obese people will be discussed later, in Chapter 5.

Two eating disorders are linked with both depression and obesity: binge eating and night eating syndrome.[8]

Binge eating syndrome

Binge eating is characterised by the rapid consumption of very large portions of food accompanied by a feeling of lack of control and inability to stop eating. Distress during eating is a feature. Eating may be secretive or solitary and it may be accompanied by feelings of self-disgust and self-hate.

Night eating syndrome

Night eating is characterised by eating more than half the daily calories after the evening meal and by feelings of guilt and anxiety when eating. Other indicators include frequent waking to eat, morning anorexia, and eating sugars and carbohydrates at inappropriate times.

If features of either of the above conditions are present, then psychological help should be sought.

Both physical and psychological ramifications may also result, not directly from medical conditions caused by obesity but by the functional impact which excess weight has on activity. Work by Larsson and Mattsson[9] and Han *et al.*[10] has found that obesity makes many activities of daily living more difficult. These include climbing stairs, bending and lifting, travelling comfortably, shopping for clothes and carrying out housework. Many of these activities have direct parallels with activities performed in the workplace.

KEY POINTS

∞   The main health consequences of obesity are diabetes and cardiovascular disease.

∞   Obesity affects almost all systems of the body, including fertility.

∞   If obesity leads to sleep apnoea, then there is an increased risk of both occupational and road traffic accidents.

∞   Obesity may result in or from eating disorders and the use of food as a comforter. Asking about eating patterns is important in evaluating the obese person.

REFERENCES

1 Packianathan I, Finer N. Medical consequences of obesity. *Clin Med.* 2003; **31** (4): 8–12.

2 Carey VJ, Walters EE, Colditz GA *et al.* Body fat distribution and risk of non-insulin-dependent diabetes mellitus in women. The Nurses' Health Study. *Am J Epidemiol.* 1997; **145**: 614–19.

3 Colditz GA, Willett WC, Rotnitzy A *et al.* Weight gain as a risk factor for clinical diabetes mellitus in women. *Ann Intern Med.* 1995; **122**: 481–86.

4 Lindberg E, Carter N, Gislason T *et al.* Role of snoring and daytime sleepiness in occupational accidents. *Am J Respir Crit Care Med.* 2001; **164**: 2031–5.

5 Teran-Santos J, Jimenez-Gomez A, Janson C. The association between sleep apnoea and the risk of road traffic accidents. Cooperative Group Burgos-Santander. *NEJM* 1999; **340**: 847–51.

6 Vanio H, Bianchini F, editors. *International Agency for Cancer Handbook of Cancer Prevention, Vol 6. Weight control and physical activity.* Lyon: IARC; 2002.

7 Kivipelto M, Ngandu T, Fratiglioni L *et al.* Obesity and vascular risk factors at midlife and the risk of dementia and Alzheimers disease. *JAMA* 2005; **62**: 1556–60.

8 Stunkard AJ, Binge-eating disorder and the night eating syndrome. In: Wadden TA, Stunkard AJ, editors. *Handbook on Obesity Treatment.* New York: Guildford Press; 2002: 107–21.

9 Larsson UE, Mattsson E. Perceived disability and observed functional limitations in obese women. *Int J Obes Res* 2001; **25**: 1705–12.

10 Han TS *et al*. X, Quality of life in relation to overweight and body fat distribution. *Am J Public Health* 1999; **88**: 1814–20.

CHAPTER 4

The workplace implications of obesity: the fit between worker and workplace

'Never eat more than you can lift.'

SIGN AT NEWCASTLE AIRPORT RESTAURANT UK, 19 MAY 2006

FITNESS FOR WORK

Obesity has significant implications for individuals, their work and their working environment. This is due to the impact of excess weight on fitness, ability to use equipment and ergonomic organisation.

An overview of the potential for impact was documented in a study undertaken in an NHS obesity clinic, which sought the views of a sample of patients on how their weight affected their working life. The ages of study participants is shown below – the majority were of working age.

Headline findings included:

▮ 17% of this population were unemployed or on incapacity benefits (state social security benefits)
▮ 79% thought their weight affected their employment and in 58% this was a negative effect
▮ 13% thought their weight affected their promotion prospects
▮ 50% had taken time off for health problems which they attributed to their weight
▮ 25% had difficulty wearing work uniforms
▮ 30% had difficulty wearing personal protective equipment.

In terms of work ability, the study sample reported:
▮ 17% had difficulty with transport in getting to work

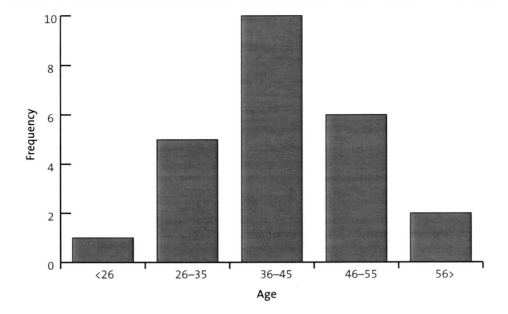

FIGURE 4.1 Age distribution of respondents to study on work implications of obesity. (From Williams NR, Malik N. Obesity and work: perceptions of a sample of patients attending an NHS obesity clinic. *Occupational Health* 2005. Reproduced with permission from *Occupational Health*.)

▌ 17% had difficulty in getting around at work
▌ 21% had problems attending training courses
▌ 13% had difficulty with the arrangement of their desk and their computer but none had difficulty actually using the keyboard.

This study supported the earlier findings of Larsson and Mattsson[1] and Han *et al.*,[2] who looked at the functional limitations of overweight and obese people and found difficulty with everyday activities such as climbing stairs and bending and lifting.

What was not studied in the previous work was the ability of individuals to respond to emergencies – in the Williams and Malik study reported above, a worrying 17% also had difficulties attending emergencies –a key part of their role in many jobs.

In looking at the potential issues around obesity and work it is useful to consider the various aspects of workability:

AEROBIC AND CARDIOVASCULAR FITNESS

A small number of jobs have specific fitness requirements and a standard of aerobic fitness is needed both at pre-employment and during the course of the job. Examples of such jobs include fire-fighters, services personnel and emergency crew on oil and gas platforms. Other groups of workers may have emergency duties as only a small part of their job and have no specific medical standard to maintain but need to be able to run to summon help (in the case of train drivers) or respond to administer treatment (paramedics, doctors and nurses).

Being obese does not, on its own, preclude someone from being physically active and many overweight and obese people can meet fitness standards. It is the obese physically inactive person who may fail or be unable to respond as required, but it should always be remembered that a physically active obese person may be, and often is, more able to cope with physical activity than a sedentary 'thinner' colleague.

The reduction in aerobic and cardiovascular fitness that accompanies excessive weight gain is due to a combination of factors. The deposition of fat in the thorax may act as a physical reason for reduced respiratory capacity and may also be associated with difficulty in wearing respiratory protective equipment – particularly important for fire-fighters and administering first-aid. General deconditioning and lack of physical exercise may occur particularly in the presence of painful hips and knee joints, and the presence of co-existing cardiovascular disease can impair cardiovascular fitness.

MOBILITY AND PHYSICAL AGILITY

The presence of back pain, knee and hip osteoarthritis can affect overall mobility both in response to emergency situations (e.g. cardiac arrests) or routine tasks (such as apprehending or restraining offenders). Osteoarthritis of the hands can lead to impaired grip (relevant in jobs involving restraint, such as prison officers or police) and size can impair physical agility.

In non-emergency situations, the reduced mobility that results from gross obesity is important, as it needs to be covered by risk assessments, particularly for emergency evacuations in event of fire in all workplaces.

ERGONOMICS

The ergonomics of obesity can be described in terms of:
- the use of routine workplace equipment
- the use of personal protective equipment
- uniforms

Routine use of workplace equipment

Obese people are larger in most of the standard ergonomic dimensions than people of normal weight but they are particularly large in abdominal girth and anterior posterior 'width'. This is important as it affects their ability to get close to their desk or workstation and to use equipment such as keyboards and fixed tools in an ergonomic way. The ergonomic ranges of common dimensions of populations which are used in furniture and workplace design were devised many years ago, when populations were much thinner. Equipment and facilities based on these ranges are likely to be woefully inadequate for the population of the 21st century. This is important particularly for the manufacture and supply of office furniture – as in the hospital study mentioned above, where 13% of respondents had difficulty sitting at a computer workstation but 0% had difficulty actually using the keyboard.[3] Obese people may have difficulty getting into and out of seats with fixed arms, and with gas-activated chairs which can be adjusted up and down – these have a weight load, which they may exceed. They may also have difficulty fitting their thighs under desks and work surfaces, even after adjusting chair height. The specific needs of larger workers needs to be sensitively considered in the ergonomic assessment process and also when offices are being planned, as larger workers are not always able to squeeze between desks and furniture in the standard arrangement of open plan offices. Insensitively managed, this could lead to personal embarrassment and humiliation, which must be avoided by designing in the needs of larger people at the start of the process.

Personal protective equipment (ppe)

The deposition of fat around the abdomen may make wearing protective equipment more difficult or less effective. Three examples of the potential difficulties faced by users of stab vests, plastic aprons and respiratory masks and equipment are outlined below.

Stab vests worn by groups such as the police need to cover the chest and abdomen but truncal obesity raises the vest and exposures the mid-abdomen. Larger vests can be worn, but there are then issues regarding overall fit and, in the case of some protective equipment, added weight and usability for the length of time the equipment needs to be worn.

Plastic aprons are worn by groups such as nurses and are provided partly to improve infection control for the benefit of staff but primarily to prevent the transfer of infection between patients. They are usually supplied for communal rather than personal use and come on a roll where each disposable apron is pulled off. Truncal obesity can enlarge the abdomen to such a degree that it is not possible to tie the apron, so it is worn hanging loose around the neck, untied. The uniform is thus exposed and could act as a conduit for infection. Embarrassment or the lack of suitably sized aprons available on order can perpetuate the problem.

Respiratory equipment, such as face masks, is designed to protect against fumes or dust but, with just a day's facial hair growth, its efficacy is reduced – as is well documented. However, what is often not appreciated is that when people put on weight, their facial contours change and masks may not fit properly or provide adequate protection. This is a difficulty in addition to the effect of the resistance, which users experience in breathing in and out when wearing masks, and the effect of fat deposition on respiratory function also seen in obesity.

Uniforms

Uniforms may be provided to portray a corporate image or a sense of togetherness, or they may have a more practical application in protection from soiling. Off-the-peg uniforms do not extend to very large sizes and there may be a need, and increased costs, of custom-made wear.

SICKNESS ABSENCE, DISABILITY AND ILL-HEALTH RETIREMENT

Studies have reported that obesity is one of the many factors which influences sickness absence. Ferrie and colleagues[4] studied over 5500 British civil servants on entry to the Whitehall study between 1985 and 1988. They took baseline anthropometric measures and questionnaire data. Sickness absence for both short (less than seven days) and medically certified (beyond seven days) spells per year were recorded. Body mass index at age 25 and baseline were examined in relation to sickness absence over the subsequent five years. Taking into account factors such as employment grade, health-related behaviour and mental and physical health indicators, the researchers concluded that:

▌ obesity was a significant predictor of short-term absence in women and
▌ both overweight and obesity were significant predictors of short-term absence in men.

With regard to longer absences:
▌ overweight and obesity were predictive for women but only obesity was predictive for men.

Another finding was that weight gain between the age of 25 and baseline was also associated with increased short- and long-term sickness absences.

Effects were much stronger in women, with a gain of more than 15 kg being associated with an excess risk for long absence of 43% but only 15% in men. When other factors were considered, this 43% reduced to 23% in the fully adjusted model.

The researchers concluded that, due to the current obesity epidemic in the industrialised world, further increases in sickness absence were likely to occur and that policy aimed at reducing sickness absence would also need to address the issues of weight and weight gain in the working population.

Finnish studies have shown that whilst body mass index is a poor predictor of death, it is a strong predictor of early work disability, which increases as body mass index increases.[5] Increased risks are due to cardiovascular and musculoskeletal diseases, but not to mental ill-health. Of all disability pensions from cardiovascular and musculoskeletal diseases, over a quarter in women and over half in men could be attributed to being overweight. Researchers concluded that although being modestly overweight had little impact on mortality, it predicted severe functional impairment and that the award of disability pensions could be prevented by effective weight management.

The impact of obesity on work limitations was reviewed by Hertz *et al.*, who found that obese workers experienced higher rates of work limitations compared to normal weight workers (6.9% vs 3.0%); obese workers also had significantly higher levels of hypertension, dyslipidaemia, diabetes and metabolic syndrome when compared to normal weight colleagues. The effect of obesity on work limitations and cardiovascular risk factors was about the same magnitude as 20 years of aging – i.e. the rate of work limitations in younger obese workers was about the same as those of normal weight middle-aged colleagues.[6]

Lifestyle is probably the most important influence on weight, but what happens when people retire and what impact is there likely to be on pensions? A Dutch study measured changes in weight and waist circumference over a five-year period in 288 male participants. The effect of retirement depended on the type of the former occupation.

Men who retired from active jobs had a greater increase in both body weight and waist circumference than did men who retired from sedentary jobs. Weight gain and waist circumference increase were associated with a reduced consumption of fruit and fibre density of diet, an increased frequency of eating breakfast and a decrease in physical activities such as cycling, walking and doing household jobs. Thus there was a clear message for active workers facing retirement who want to claim their pension for as long as possible.[7]

DO SOME JOBS MAKE PEOPLE OBESE?

There is no conclusive or persuasive evidence linking specific occupations with obesity, as no longitudinal studies of groups of workers have been undertaken. Anecdotally, physicians working in obesity clinics have reported over-representation of patients working in catering – particularly chefs, waiters and school catering staff. This should not be surprising, given the ready availability of food during their working day. Other groups who have reported increased weight after starting work are call centre operators, who spend most of the day sitting, and shift workers, who often have no access to healthy food and cannot easily leave the workplace to make healthier choices.

The link between specific jobs and work organisation and weight gain requires research to identify the interventions that could be introduced to prevent weight gain in these occupational groups.

HOW OPEN ARE ISSUES RELATING TO OBESITY?

Obesity is a sensitive issue and, from the Birmingham study, certainly from the perspective of the obese employees, not one which is often discussed. We need to encourage better understanding and appreciation of the potential difficulties faced by obese workers, from the amount of additional space they need to move around an open plan office, to their particular needs so as to avoid embarrassing team-building exercises which bring their weight into focus.

One of the most difficult areas is that of company image. Because obesity is common, and likely to be even more so in the future, business needs to start to think now about how they will manage issues of image if they are in an image-sensitive business sector. A media frenzy was recently caused by a human resources manager at a health club company who sent an internal memo to staff on the 'impact of larger employees' affecting the company's image. This sort of insensitivity (and hypocrisy, given the likely size of many of its target customers) can damage the company in the eyes of both its consumers and its employees.

BOX 4.1 Difficulties obese people have reported

- getting to work
- getting around at work
- attending training courses
- attending emergency drills
- using standard office desks
- using personal protective equipment.

(From Williams NR, Malik N. Obesity and work: perceptions of a sample of patients attending an NHS obesity clinic. *Occupational Health*. October 2005. Reproduced with permission from *Occupational Health*.)

KEY POINTS

Obesity may impact on:

- ∞ cardiovascular and aerobic fitness
- ∞ the use of personal protective equipment
- ∞ the use of uniforms
- ∞ the ability to mount an emergency response.

REFERENCES

1 Larsson UE, Mattsson E. Perceived disability and observed functional limitations in obese women. *Int J Obes Res* 2001; **25**: 1705–12.

2 Han TS *et al*. X, Quality of life in relation to overweight and body fat distribution. *Am J Public Health* 1999; **88**: 1814–20.

3 Williams NR, Malik N. Obesity and work: perceptions of a sample of patients attending an NHS obesity clinic. *Occupational Health*. October 2005.

4 Ferrie JE, Kivimaki M, Head J. *Weight and weight gain: implications for sickness absence in British civil servants over a five-year period from the late 1980s. Track 3 work-related health problems and healthcare needs*. www.eupha.org.html/2005

5 Rissanen A, Heliovaara M, Knekt P *et al*. Risk of disability and mortality due to overweight in a Finnish population. *BMJ* 1990; **301** (6756): 835–7.

6 Hertz RP, Unger AN, McDonald M *et al*. The impact of obesity on work limitations and cardiovascular risk factors in the US workforce. *J Occup Environ Med*. 2005; **46** (12): 1196–203.

7 Nooyens AC, Vissacher TL, Schuit AJ *et al*. Effects of retirement on lifestyle in relation to changes in weight and waist circumference in Dutch men: a prospective study. *Public Health Nutr*. 2005: **8** (8): 1266–74.

CHAPTER 5

Prejudice and discrimination in employment and healthcare

'In a society that all too often confuses "slim" with "beautiful" or "good", morbid obesity can present formidable barriers to employment.'

BRUCE SELYA (PRESIDING JUDGE IN *COOK VS RHODE ISLAND DEPARTMENT OF MENTAL HEALTH*)

CHALLENGES: PREJUDICE AND DISCRIMINATION

In considering obese people in the workplace it is important to recognise that obesity, along with height, is probably one of the last bastions of discrimination. In Europe, legislation against discrimination on the grounds of:

▮ gender
▮ race
▮ sexual orientation and
▮ religion

already exists, with age discrimination the latest, implemented in the UK in October 2006.

Obesity is rarely considered an issue in diversity programmes and training, yet evidence suggests that discrimination and prejudice against obese people remains common across healthcare and business.

Some of the most important work has been done on the effect on salary of a person being obese. Saport and Halpern investigated the effect of being overweight and of being thin on the salaries of lawyers.[1] In examining the salaries and personal measurements of respondents to the 1984 National Lawyer Survey, they found that overweight and thin male lawyers were paid less than normal weight individuals. The same was not found for women. It has been long established that physical appearance is important to how people are treated. Even going back to babies, research has shown that different treatment is given by mothers for children as young as three months of age depending on their attractiveness.[2] School-age children who are attractive are rated higher academically by their parents when compared to less good-looking but equally competent peers.[3] Adults presume that better-looking children have better personalities, are better behaved and more honest.[4] All of these are assumptions based on attractiveness, and within the Western world thinness is equated with attractiveness and obesity with unattractiveness.

This has wide-ranging impact on all stages of life and on opportunity – even to the extent of likelihood of access to higher education, which was found to be greater in the attractive.[5]

This attribution of special or better qualities is known as the 'halo' effect of attractiveness, and even in professions unlikely to value physical appearance attractiveness ratings can predict future promotion. This is graphically seen in the US, where one panel assessed cadets at West Point military academy for attractiveness and a separate panel assessed intelligence and ability to lead. Attractive cadets scored most highly in their leadership potential and their attractiveness rating predicted their rank several years later.[6]

Weight is one of the most important determinants of attractiveness, but it is the ratio of height to weight which is thought to be most important.[7] A person's weight is thought to reflect many aspects of their character, such as their motivation, willingness to work, ambition, personal control and discipline. This can influence employers' decisions regarding recruitment, promotion and salary.

The literature suggests that short people and unattractive people do not fare as well in the workplace as do tall and attractive people. This comes from both laboratory experiments and field studies. Worryingly, physical attractiveness has been found to affect interviewers' judgements when they assess curriculum vitaes of potential managers.[8]

In a detailed study, Saporta and Halpern used eight different models to explore the impact of weight on lawyers' salaries. They found that in each model, there was some evidence that being overweight had a negative effect on salary. In a separate study, it was also found that there was some evidence that both overweight and underweight females were less likely to have jobs that required face-to-face interaction with the public.[9]

These studies suggest subtle and sometimes not-so-subtle prejudices and discrimination based on weight within the employment setting, but more overt prejudice occurs. In a landmark legal ruling, *Cook vs Rhode Island Department of Mental Health, Retardation and Hospitals*, the hospital employer was found to have violated the 1973 *Rehabilitation Act* which prohibited disability discrimination by federal bodies when they refused to employ an obese applicant.[10] The court rejected arguments that morbid obesity was not a disability because it was a changeable condition within the person's control. The ruling also applied to claims brought under the *Americans with Disabilities Act*, meaning that private sector employers could also be charged with discrimination against obese people.

And legislation is much needed. Roe and Eickwort[11] found in a survey of 81 employers (including HR professionals) that 15.9% of employers held the view that obese applicants should be barred from employment and 43.9% believed that obesity was a valid medical reason for not employing a person. Studies have suggested that obese people are perceived to possess negative traits, such as being less conscientious (more lazy),[12] less self-disciplined and self-controlled,[13] less able to get on with customers and fellow workers,[14] more likely to have an emotional problem,[5] and less competent than their slimmer counterparts.[13, 14]

Professor Mark Roehling, Professor in the Department of Management at Western Michigan University in the US, has undertaken pioneering research into the effects of obesity in employment. From his many studies he has concluded that 'overall the evidence of consistent, significant discrimination against overweight employees is sobering'.[15] He found that overweight people were subject to discrimination in employment decisions based on body weight; they were also stereotyped as being emotionally impaired and socially handicapped and as possessing negative personality traits. The wages of mildly obese white women were 5.9% lower than standard weight counterparts and very obese women had wages 24.1% lower. Men only experienced penalties at the very highest weight levels.

Other studies have shown discrimination in recruitment and employee discharge, for not only do overweight and obese people face prejudice and have more difficulty in getting a job, and receive less pay when in it, but they are more likely to be selected for redundancy[15, 16] and to have specific jobs denied them.[17]

An indication of the depth of prejudice against obese people is seen in the conclusions drawn by Kennedy and Homant following their research. They found that overweight job applicants were treated more harshly by employers when applying for work than ex-felons or individuals with a past history of mental ill-health.[18]

Looking at a summary of cases taken under federal law in the US,[15] it is noticeable that the occupations of individuals fall into two broad groups: those who have a weight or fitness standard for the job – such as police officers, flight attendants and fire-fighters – and those who have work which may have contributed to their obesity – restaurant managers, delivery drivers, office workers. It is members of these latter occupational groups who, at least according to litigation, require most attention in workplace weight management programmes.

But perceptions of overweight and obese people are not confined to human resource and management professionals. Healthcare workers have been reported to believe that obese people are less intelligent, less likely to have friends and more lazy than people of normal weight.

Surprisingly a study of dieticians in the UK reported mixed attitudes to overweight and obese people. Although generally neutral to positive, the negative attitudes included a belief that these patients had reduced self-esteem, sexual attractiveness and health. Dieticians rated obese people more negatively than overweight people.[19] In a further study, this time of doctors, 67% of respondents surveyed felt that obese people lacked self-control, 39% thought they were lazy and 34% that they were sad.[20]

In a separate study, involving 24 obese patients attending an outpatient weight management clinic in Birmingham, UK, only 42% of patients who completed the questionnaire felt that their GP was sympathetic towards them and their efforts to lose weight, while 18% felt that GPs were neutral and 42% unsympathetic. The findings were not much different for practice nurses (46% sympathetic), although they were often not even consulted.[21]

But what of the workers? Do they feel disadvantaged and discriminated against? Again, there is little research that helps to answer the question but a study in the US did look at perceived discrimination and psychological well-being in relation to body weight. Compared to normal weight people, people with a body mass index of 35 or more reported more institutional and day-to-day interpersonal discrimination. Professional workers were more likely to report discrimination and interpersonal mistreatment than non-professionals. Obese workers reported lower levels of self-acceptance. This study offered further support for the stigma of obesity and the negative effect of self-identity on life chances.[22] Responses reported in the Birmingham study give us some insight on the situation in the UK, where the stigma may not be so great or so readily perceived.[21]

Of the 24 patients interviewed:
- 79% felt that their weight affected their employment (for 58%, this was a negative effect)
- 38% felt their weight impaired their ability to get a job
- 13% felt it affected likelihood of promotion and
- 17% felt it affected their ability to attend certain types of training courses.

(Responses are expressed as a percentage of total respondents.)

Other headline findings included:
- line managers were perceived to be more likely to be neutral or unsympathetic to an employee's issues around obesity than they were to be sympathetic but
- colleagues were more likely to be sympathetic (*see below*).

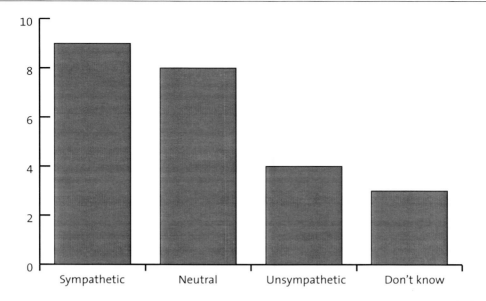

FIGURE 5.1 Perceived attitudes towards obese work colleagues. (From Williams NR, Malik N. Obesity and work: perceptions of a sample of patients attending an NHS obesity clinic. *Occupational Health*. October. Reproduced with permission from *Occupational Health*.)

HR professionals in the UK

Compared to the US, relatively little research has been undertaken in the UK on the views of human resources managers and officers, but a study published by *Personnel Today* in October 2005 contains some worrying similarities with US findings.

Headline figures, from a survey of over 2000 HR professionals, included:

- 93% said they would choose a 'normal' weight person over an obese applicant with the same qualifications and experience
- 47% thought obesity negatively affected employee output
- 30% thought obesity was a valid medical reason for not employing someone
- 75% said their organisation was doing little or nothing to tackle the issue and 69% said obesity was not discussed in their workplace
- 11% thought employers could fairly dismiss someone because they were obese and
- 12% said obese people were unsuitable for client-facing roles.

(Thomas D. Fattism is the last bastion of employee discrimination. *Personnel Today*, 25 October 2005.)

IMPACT ON ACCESS TO HEALTHCARE

We have already discussed the many co-morbidities which exist with obesity. Many of these have well-recognised and available treatments, but recent decisions on the allocation of resources mean that obese patients do not always have the same access to such services as thinner patients. This has an impact on their sickness absence and any applications for ill-health retirement as, if the treatment is not available, they will remain disabled and unable to work effectively.

One example is the decision by some primary care organisations in England to exclude people with a BMI of over 30 from hip and knee replacements. It could be argued that for someone who was obese and had poor mobility, the greatest benefit would be a joint replacement that allowed them to exercise and become active again. But the decision by East Suffolk primary care organisations (PCTs) was justified by suggesting that the outcome for such patients was poorer than for patients who weighed less.

There was no public outcry in defence of the needs of obese patients to receive treatment, as there would have been, with a letter-writing campaign and inches of media coverage, had a drug been denied to cancer sufferers. But the decision by East Suffolk PCTs becomes more interesting when it transpires that a study carried out by the University of Southampton showed that having a BMI in excess of 28 *did not* predict a decline in physical function, vitality or mental health in patients who underwent surgery. Instead, the reporting of pain in multiple joints at the start of the study was the critical predictor of success. The authors concluded 'you should not deny surgery to an obese person because you think surgery will not do them any good' (quote from Professor Cyrus Cooper, Professor of Rheumatology, University of Southampton. Published in *Pulse* 4 May 2006). Similar decisions on access to healthcare have been suggested for in-vitro fertilisation (Should obese women have IVF? *GP* 8 September 2006) and breast reduction surgery (Wales sets BMI cut-off for cosmetic breast ops. *Doctor* 16 May 2006).

Healthcare practitioners and employers need to be aware of the potential for discrimination at all levels within the workplace, from recruitment to dismissal, promotion to training opportunities and management of absence when health-care is denied.

The literature review can be summarised as identifying significant discrimination against overweight and obese individuals at several stages of the employment process and beyond. Employers may feel they are justified in not recruiting obese people because of the ergonomic costs, raised sickness absence and greater healthcare costs. However, personal motivation, talent and skills can be overlooked when prejudice exists. The increased numbers of obese people both as employees and customers might have been expected to change attitudes and long-standing prejudices, but this has yet to appear in studies. But this is more than just an upsetting issue which has significant implications for employment;

it also affects self-esteem, which is pivotal to health behaviour changes. Low self-esteem can deter people from exercising, seeking medical help and managing their own health effectively.

IS THE CUSTOMER ALWAYS RIGHT?

If an overweight or obese employee meets the job specifications and is wholly competent in carrying out the tasks required, then should negative reactions from customers affect that employee's job? How should an employer react if repeated customer comments suggest it is inappropriate, for example, for a fitness trainer in a gym to be overweight or for a slimming consultant to be less than of normal or low weight? There are clearly ethical issues for employers if they are to treat employees with fairness and respect in how they deal with some comments.

Employers need to be aware, however, that women are often perceived to be more unattractive when mildly overweight than are correspondingly mildly overweight men. Overweight women have been found to receive less attractive job assignments than overweight men[17] and even mildly obese women earn significantly less than women of normal weight, yet mildly obese men are not so disadvantaged when compared to their normal weight counterparts.[23, 24, 25]

There are ethnic differences, too – African Americans and Hispanics were found in one study to express a preference for heavier body types and were less concerned by bigger people; it was the Anglo Americans who preferred lighter-weight and smaller-sized people.[26]

In the weight-conscious US, where freedom is a much-discussed human right, anti-obesity discrimination is present in only two states – Michigan and California. In Europe, discrimination against obese people is only illegal in Italy. We have a long way to go to make obese people equal in society and in employment opportunities.

KEY POINTS

- ∞ Policies and procedures, payment and reward systems need to recognise the negative assumptions and prejudices which some individuals hold for obese people.

- ∞ Diversity training and diversity awareness needs to specifically consider the issue of appearance and body size and shape, not just age, gender, sexuality and race.

- ∞ The social acceptability of making negative comments and assumptions about obese people is pervasive and needs to be managed out of business – as have already similar comments and assumptions of a racial or gender-specific nature.

QUOTES FROM OBESE WORKERS

We had to wear company business attire, jacket, blouse and skirt. I wore high heels with my suit. One colleague wanted to know how my 'little bitty ankles and little bitty heels on those shoes held up my big old body'. I asked her how her little bitty butt held up her big fat mouth . . .

The most important thing for all people to realise is that fat people know they're fat. They don't need anyone mentioning it to them or asking 'should you eat that?' or whatever.

Colleagues make comments about exercising more, eating less etc. It still amazes me that they feel they have the right to tell me how to eat or exercise! I would never tell someone with cancer how they should live.

The major concern I have always had was when meeting in a conference room or cafeteria or staff room to always have chairs that have no arms on them. It is highly offensive for a large person to have to squeeze into a chair they know they cannot fit into. And then to have to sit there for an hour or so with their circulation being cut off.

My employer is wonderful. When I was hired, the HR director ordered a larger size office chair before I started my job so that when I arrived it was there. Now that's considerate.

RECENT CASE

The Sunday Times reported, on 19 November 2006, the case of Indian Airlines and the issue of the weight of its air hostesses. It quotes:

A group of air hostesses has vowed to fight for lost wages after being grounded by the state run airline Indian. The cabin crew, who were suspended for being between 1 lb and 7 lb over the airline's specific weight limit, accuse Indian of trying to replace them with skinnier models, but the airline says that is not true. 'This is an issue about fitness not image,' said the company lawyer Rupinder Singh Suri.

REFERENCES

1 Saporta I, Halpern JJ. Being different can hurt: effects of deviation from physical norms on lawyers' salaries. *Industrial Relations* 2002; **41**: 442–66.
2 Langlois JH. From the eye of the beholder to behavioural reality: development of

social behaviours and social relations as a function of attractiveness. In: Herman CP, Zanna MP, Higgins ET, editors. *Physical Appearance Stigma and Social Behaviour: the Ontario Symposium.* Hillsdale, NJ: Lawrence Erlbaum Associates, 1986; **3**: 23–51.

3 Lerner RM, Lerner JV. Effects of age, sex and physical attractiveness on children's peer relations, academic performance and elementary school adjustment. *Dev Psychol.* 1977; **13**: 585–90.

4 Dion K. Physical attractiveness and evaluation of children's transgressions. *J Pers Soc Psychol.* 1972; **24**: 207–13.

5 Clifford MM, Walster E. The effect of physical attractiveness on teacher expectations. *Sociol Educ.* 1973; 5: 201–9.

6 Mazur A. Military rank attainment of a West Point class: effects of cadets' physical features. *Am J Sociol.* 1984; **90** (1): 125–50.

7 Patzer GL. *Physical Attractiveness Phenomena.* New York: Plenum Press; 1985.

8 Dipboye R, Fromkin HL, Willback K. Relative importance of applicant sex, attractiveness and scholastic standing in evaluation of job applicants resumes. *J Appl Psychol.* 1975; **60**: 39–43.

9 Quinn RP. Physical deviance and occupational mistreatment: the short, the fat and the ugly. Masters thesis. University of Michigan. Ann Arbor; 1978.

10 *Cook vs Rhode Island Department of Mental Health, Retardation and Hospitals.* CA 1, No. 93–1093; 22 November 1993.

11 Roe DA, Eickwort KR. Relationships between obesity and associated health factors with low employment among low-income women. *J Am Med Women's Assoc.* 1976; **31**: 193–204.

12 Larkin JC, Pines HA. No fat persons need apply: experimental studies of the overweight stereotype and hiring preference. *Sociol Work Occup.* 1979; **6**: 312–27.

13 Klesges RC, Klem ML, Hanson CL *et al.* The effects of applicants' health status and qualifications on simulated hiring decisions. *Int J Obes.* 1990; **14**: 527–35.

14 Klassen ML, Jasper CR, Harris RJ. The role of physical appearance in managerial decisions. *J Bus Psychol.* 1990; **8**: 181–98.

15 Roehling M. Weight based discrimination in employment: psychological and legal aspects, *Personnel Psychology* 1999; **52**: 969–1016.

16 Roehling MV. Weight discrimination in the American workplace: ethical issues and analysis. *J Bus Ethics.* 2002; **40**: 177–89.

17 Bellizzi JA, Klassen ML, Belonax JJ. Stereotypical beliefs about overweight and smoking and decision making in assignments to sales territories. *Percept Mot Skills* 1989; **69**: 419–29.

18 Kennedy DB, Homant RJ. Personnel managers and the stigmatised employee. *Journal of Employment Counselling* 1984; **21**: 89–94.

19 Harvey EL, Summerbell CD, Kirk SFL *et al.* Dieticians' views of overweight and obese people and reported management practices. *J Hum Nutr Diet.* 2002; **15** (5): 331–47.

20 Price JH, Desmond SM, Krol RA. Family practice physicians' beliefs, attitudes and practices regarding obesity. *Am J Prevent Med.* 1987; **3** (6): 339–45.

21 Williams NR, Malik N. Obesity and work: perceptions of a sample of patients attending an NHS obesity clinic. *Occupational Health* October 2005.

22 Carr D, Friedman MA. Is obesity stigmatizing? Body weight, perceived discrimination and psychological well being in the United States. *J Health Soc Behav.* 2005; **46** (3): 244–59.

23 Maranto CL, Stenoien AF. Weight discrimination: a multi disciplinary analysis. Industrial Relations Researchers Associations Annual Conference, Chicago, US, 1997.

24 Pagan JA, Davila A. Obesity, occupational attainment and earnings. *Soc Sci Q.* 1997; **78**: 756–70.

25 Register CA, Williams DR. Wage effects of obesity among young workers. *Soc Sci Q.* 1990; **71**: 130–41.

26 Jackson LA, McGill OD. Body type preference and body characteristics associated with attractive and unattractive bodies by African Americans and Anglo Americans. *Sex Roles.* 1996; **35**: 295–307.

CHAPTER 6

Current management of obesity

> 'Quod me nutrit me destuit.' (What nourishes
> me also destroys me.)

In order to manage obesity effectively in the workplace setting, it is essential to understand current management approaches to engaging and influencing workers and ensuring that there is a common consistent message about what works and what does not.

This chapter will deal with advice on nutrition and physical activity which individuals need to appreciate and action in order to lose weight and reduce their personal risks of heart disease, diabetes, hypertension and other health issues. In very simplistic terms, obesity usually results over a long period of time due to an imbalance between the number of calories taken into the body and the number of calories burnt, both by body processes and by physical activity. There are many influences on this balance – genetic, familial and hormonal – but getting nutrition and physical activity right will lead to a reduction in weight and improvement in health risk factors.

NUTRITION

Most people are not aware of how many calories they consume or the fat, sugar and calorie content of their food. Several conventional diets advocated calorie counting; this suits some people but not all and calorie-counted diets were no more or less successful than any others. Individuals need to be given specific advice on what is right for them if they have special dietary needs or co-existing medical conditions which require restricted diets. However, everyone needs to know some basics of nutrition and would benefit from the following advice which are taken from the Department of Health's *Choosing a Better Diet: a food and health action plan*.[1]

Diet composition

▌ Try to eat at least 5 portions of fruit and vegetables every day (studies suggest the average consumed is currently only currently 2.8 portions per day)
▌ Decrease added sugar to 11% energy intake (currently 12.7%)
▌ Decrease total fat to 35% of energy intake (currently 35.3%)
▌ Decrease energy intake from saturated fat to 11% (currently 13.3%)
▌ Decrease salt to 6 g per day (currently 9.5 g)
▌ Increase dietary fibre intake to 18 g per day (currently 13.8 g)

Note: fruit and vegetables
▌ Ensure *at least* 5 portions of fruit and vegetables per day but not including potatoes.

The above recommendations don't really help in the practical world of advising on healthy diet, but they can be met by following the basic rules:
▌ base your meals on starchy foods (bread, pasta, rice etc.)
▌ eat lots of fruit and vegetables
▌ eat more fish
▌ cut down on saturated fat and sugar
▌ try to eat less salt
▌ drink plenty of water
▌ don't skip breakfast.

Food labelling

If success is going to be achieved at weight loss and weight maintenance, then we need to understand more about what is in our food and that means understanding more about food labelling. The basics are summarised below.

Fat

▌ Products containing 20 g or more of fat per 100 g are high in fat, and 5 g of saturated fat or more per 100 g is a lot.
▌ Products containing 3 g or less of fat per 100 g are low in fat, and 1 g saturated fat or less per 100 g is a small amount.

Sugar

▌ Products containing more than 10 g sugars per 100 g are high in sugar.
▌ Products containing less than 2 g sugars per 100 g are low in sugar.

For more information on deciding on content of food, see the Food Standards Agency (FSA) website (www.eatwell.gov.uk). The FSA introduced a new traffic light system of labelling in January 2007. It aims to provide customers with a simple colour-coded method of selecting healthy foods. Food manufacturers and some major food retailers have also launched their own labelling systems which are quite different, making the job of the conscientious consumer almost impossible and increasing the need for expert guidance.

Portion size

It is not only what we eat that is important but also the size of the portion. One way of deciding how much to eat is to follow the guidance in the FSA's 'balance of good health' (BOGH), which divides food into five groups:

a   fruit and vegetables
b   bread, other cereals and potatoes
c   milk and dairy foods
d   meat, fish and alternatives
e   foods containing fat and sugar.

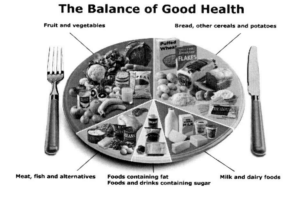

FIGURE 6.1 The balance of good health. (Reproduced with permission of the Food Standards Agency.)

Foods from the largest groups (a etc.) should be eaten most often and foods from the smallest groups (e etc.), eaten less often. The guide is shaped like a dinner plate, which has been designed to make healthy eating simpler to understand and interpret. It is necessary to achieve this balance between the various food groups at each meal but it is recommended that it be applied to food eaten over a day or even a week.

The aim of the BOGH is to illustrate the types and proportion of foods which make up a well-balanced and healthy diet. It seeks to encourage people to choose a variety of foods from the first four groups every day. The fifth group – foods containing fat and sugar – are not essential to a healthy diet but add choice and palatability. Further guidance on the BOGH can be found at www.good.gov.uk/multimedia/pdfs/bghbooklet.pdf

Overall philosophy

Diets fail because people do not adhere to them. The philosophy now is not for people to diet but to make lifestyle changes which mount up over time. Just as it is the case that an extra 100 calories per day leads to a weight increase of 5 kg per year, so a 100-calorie-a-day deficit leads to a 5 kg loss.

The aim is to devise an eating regime that produces a daily deficit of 600 calories, leading to a weekly loss of 4200 calories. This is the equivalent of .45–.68 kg fat (each pound of fat lost requires a daily calorie deficit of 3300 calories). This level of weight loss is often too slow for individuals used to losing half a stone (3.2 kg) in a week, but this is the speed and approach that leads to long-standing weight loss and weight loss maintenance. Fad diets often lead to weight gain and rebound effects after only a few weeks or months.

Usually the average female needs around 2000 calories per day and the average male, 2500 calories per day. But these figures do not take into account the age and level of physical activity which a person is involved in. Several methods are available to calculate daily calorie levels needed. One has been developed by Kosasek et al.[2] Another is the Harris-Benedict formula found in nutrition textbooks.

The loss of .45–.68 kg per week is big enough to make a difference in a matter of weeks, but small enough not to cause hunger or the body to compensate for an acute calorie reduction. The easier it is to eat food that is filling and that satisfies hunger, the more likely the person is to keep to the regime. Many diets fail because they are extreme and people become hungry, break the rules then see no point in continuing.

Knowing what workers know

Many workers will be experts on diets because they have tried them all. In the workplace setting it is important to be aware of some of the more popular diets so that good foods and bad diets can be highlighted. A brief resume of several very popular diets is included in Appendix 3.

What the evidence says

We know that the key to weight loss is essentially a reduction of calories taken in over calories burnt off. We know that fat provides the most calories per gram, so if we are to create a calorie deficit we need to reduce fat intake. However, we also know the importance of not excluding fats and carbohydrates, but instead having a balanced diet.

We know that having lost weight, further weight reduction often plateaus and becomes harder. This is because energy requirements are greater for someone of a heavier weight and, when weight is lost, the daily calorie intake calculation has to be re-done and a lower level of calories consumed per day in order to lose further weight.

PHYSICAL ACTIVITY

The Department of Health, in its document *Choosing Activity: a physical activity action plan*,[3] states that increased physical activity helps in the prevention and management of over 20 conditions including:

- coronary heart disease
- diabetes
- cancer
- mental ill-health.

As well, increased physical activity reduces the risk of developing:

- osteoporosis, back pain and osteoarthritis.

Current guidance[3] for physical activity is that all adults undertake at least five sessions of 30 minutes or more exercise per week. More specific guidance is available for people with specific conditions. The recommended levels can be achieved through short bursts of exercise of 10 minutes each or 30 minutes in one period. The exercise should be enough to make someone slightly breathless but still able to talk. Practically, however, it suggests that most people will need to undertake at least 45–60 minutes exercise per day to prevent obesity with today's lifestyles.

For children and young adults, at least 60 minutes exercise of at least moderate intensity each day of the week is advised, and on at least two occasions during the week the activity should improve bone health and muscle strength and flexibility.

Another, perhaps better known, recommendation is that adults should walk at least 10 000 steps per day, preferably 15 000. But in reality, when all sources of activity are considered, only about 37% of men and 24% of women meet these recommendations.[4]

Its important to recognise that physical activity can be of any type – an intensive aerobic workout, a gentle run in the park, a brisk walk with the dog. Overall, physical activity has several advantages for weight loss and weight maintenance.

- It builds lean muscle bulk.
- It releases endorphins, which lift mood.
- It burns calories, but not as many as most people would like.

What the evidence says

There is a lot we don't know about physical activity, including exactly how it compares with diet as a means of weight loss, but there is evidence in three important areas.

▪ Physical activity programmes in the workplace are successful.
▪ Physical activity helps keep weight off.
▪ Physical activity has many other benefits, too, as outlined above.

Guidance for healthcare professionals and patients has now been produced by the UK Department of Health and is contained in the document *Obesity Care Pathway and Your Weight and Your Health*, published 4 May 2006 and available to download free of charge from the Department of Health website, www.dh.gov.uk/publicationsandstatistics

COMMERCIAL WEIGHT LOSS PROGRAMMES

The role and value of commercial organisations such as Weight Watchers, Rosemary Conley and Slimming World has recently been discussed. Referrals to these types of groups has been shown to be effective for some types of patients. Researchers offered free attendance at a local Slimming World group for 12 weeks to patients with a BMI of 30 or more who were members of two GP practices in Derby. Two-thirds completed the 12-week course and the average weight loss was 5.4 kg, 6.4% of baseline body weight. One-third of participants chose to fund a further 12 attendances themselves. Their average weight loss over 24 weeks was 11.1 kg or 11.3% of baseline body weight. Certainly both groups demonstrated that, for those who stayed the course, weight loss of amounts significant enough to enhance health could be achieved (www.sciencedirect.com accessed 18 August 2006).

MEDICAL MANAGEMENT OF OBESITY

If lifestyle advice does not lead to significant weight loss, then the use of medication maybe indicated. Although this would not be prescribed in the occupational health and workplace setting, it is important that practitioners who are planning and delivering weight loss programmes are aware of the additional medical assistance which can be accessed.

There are four drugs currently licensed for the treatment of obesity.

1 Orlistat (trade name: Xenical; manufacturer, Roche), which reduces the absorption of dietary fat.
2 Sibutramine (trade name: Reductil; manufacturer, Abbott), which enhances satiety – i.e. makes a person feel fuller having eaten smaller portions of food.
3 Drugs which act to fill the stomach and so produce a 'full' feeling through

local action in the stomach. There have been few studies of the effectiveness of these agents and so they will not be discussed further here.

4   The latest drug, Rimonabant (trade name: Accomplia; manufacturer, Sanofi-Aventis), which acts on endocannabinoid receptors in the brain, affecting hunger centres.

Orlistat

Orlistat (Xenical; Roche) is a pancreatic and gastric lipase inhibitor, which reduces the amount of fat absorbed into the body. It is taken three times per day but must be used in conjunction with a low-fat diet or else the risk of side effects increases. If fatty foods are eaten, then unpleasant oily diarrhoea and urgency to defecate results. Patients can now either buy Orlistat over the counter or obtain it on prescription from their doctor. It can be taken for several years but is not a replacement for lifestyle improvement. Consequently, when it is prescribed, advice on a healthy diet and increased physical activity is reiterated. Only about 2% of the drug is actually absorbed into the body and it produces weight loss by inhibiting the breakdown and absorption of fat, thereby reducing calorie intake. There have been theoretical concerns that, with long-term use, there may be deficiencies of fat-soluble vitamins, but no evidence is yet available.

(*Disclaimer*: this is not meant to replace medical advice, which should always be sought before medication is taken, or embarking on a diet.)

Sibutramine

Sibutramine (Reductil; Abbott) is a centrally acting satiety enhancer – i.e. it gives the feeling of being full or satiated. One very important point is that it is not an appetite suppressant, and it is very different from the older appetite suppressants which were prescribed years ago. Sibutramine makes the patient feel fuller on a smaller portion of food and so reduces their calorie intake. It is contraindicated in the presence of depression and hypertension and, in the early stages of treatment, both pulse and blood pressure need to be measured frequently. It is particularly suitable for patients who have difficulties with the size of the portions of food that they eat, as it aims to retrain the appetite to be satisfied with less. It can be continued for a maximum of 12 months provided patients meet certain goals for weight loss.

Both Orlistat and Sibutramine have been recommended by NICE for use with obese patients and with those who are less overweight but who have co-existing disease.[5,6] Studies have shown that the medication can help to achieve 10% weight loss that can be maintained for two years. Maximum benefit is gained by six months after the therapy is started. Patients who successfully lose weight not only become more mobile but also show improvement in metabolic factors such as blood glucose and blood pressure. The two medications, however, should not be used together.

Rimonabant

This medication (Accomplia; Sanofi-Aventis) has recently become available. It has a different mechanism of action than either Orlistat or Sibutramine in that it affects the cannabinoid receptors to alter the parts of the brain that regulate hunger and cravings for substances such as alcohol, food and cigarettes. It also works on both the adrenal gland and the sympathetic nerves. In trials, Accomplia was compared with placebo and subjects were placed on a calorie-controlled diet (600 calories per day deficit). Two levels of drug dosage were compared with placebo. Of the 920 subjects who completed the study protocol, those on the higher dose of the drug lost the most weight (5 kg more than placebo) and lost more centimetres (7.6 cm more than placebo) off their waists. Risk factors for heart disease such as HDL cholesterol also improved. The side-effects reported were nausea, dizziness and diarrhoea. However, caution is needed as there were no changes or improvements in blood pressure, total cholesterol or heart rate.

NICE has recently reviewed its guidance on obesity and on the role of drugs and surgery for both adults and children. Up-to-date NICE guidance can be found at www.nice.org.

SURGICAL MANAGEMENT OF OBESITY

The use of surgery in obese patients is now mainstream therapy in both the US and Europe. If lifestyle advice and drug therapy does not achieve adequate weight reduction, then consideration may be given to one of the several types of surgery which have been evaluated. This is because, untreated, the mortality and morbidity of gross obesity is high. Indeed it has been estimated that, untreated, only one in seven obese people will have a normal life expectancy.

In the last 10 years, the National Institutes for Health (NIH) in the US, the National Institute for Clinical Excellence (NICE) in the UK and the Scottish Collegiate Guidelines Network (SIGN) in Scotland have all suggested surgery as effective treatment for selected patients with morbid (i.e. BMI > 40 kg/m^2) obesity.

Guidelines, which vary slightly, have been produced by organisations such as NICE and the International Federation for the Surgery of Obesity (IFSO). The types of obesity sufferer identified by these groups are people either with BMIs > 40 or with BMI > 35 and co-morbidities such as diabetes, an age range of between 18 and 55 years, the failure of medical management and the presence of an acceptable operative risk.

Evaluation of the effectiveness of obesity surgery has concluded that not only does it improve biological risk factors such as high blood pressure and diabetes, the latter which it can even cure,[7] but it also improves abnormal lipid profiles and reduces sleep apnoea and musculoskeletal problems.[8] Specifically in relation to employment, studies have shown improved employment rates of post-surgery patients.[8]

Surgery for obesity is not new. For many years jaw wiring was popular, particularly in the US, but its results were neither impressive nor sustained. Early highly invasive gastric surgery also resulted in frequent morbidity and gastrointestinal upset and so fell from favour. The current range of surgical options generally have lower morbidity and mortality than their predecessors and are more acceptable on grounds of efficacy, potential side-effects, safety and cost.

Basically, surgery is of two types, either reducing the size of the stomach or bypassing the intestines and so producing reduced absorption of nutrients.

Laparoscopic banding

The insertion of a gastric band through a small incision in the abdomen is a day-case procedure which seeks to make a smaller pocket at the top of the stomach and so make patients feel full on small amounts of food. The size of the aperture through which food can pass can be adjusted to make a pouch as large or as small as needed. Insertion of a band has been reported to lead to the loss of 22.6–27.2 kg of weight, which is then maintained for at least six years.[9]

Vertical banded gastroplasty

This is a more invasive procedure, carrying higher post-operative risks, in which the stomach capacity is reduced. In 1996 SIGN advised that this form of surgery was preferable to gastric bypass surgery as this technique was capable of producing substantial improvements and weight loss even in patients with extremely high BMIs.[10]

Gastric bypass

This is the most major type of surgery, involving a longer hospitalisation and a higher rate of complications. The abdomen is opened and a procedure performed whereby food is diverted from the stomach to the lower intestines, thus producing reduced absorption of food and nutrients. Possible side-effects include constipation, headache, dumping (an unpleasantly fast transit time through the gut when food is eaten) and intolerance to dairy products. Patients may become anaemic, vitamin deficient and develop hernias in the abdominal wall scar.

The results of the more complex surgery are impressive – data from over 14 000 patients on the International Register of Obesity Surgery show that at 12 months, vertical banded gastroplasty and gastric bypass patients show a mean loss of 53% and 72% excess weight respectively, with an operative mortality of 0.17% and with 93% of patients experiencing no morbidity.[11] NICE has produced guidance on the indications for surgery in the UK[12] and has further extended its recommendations for surgery in children (www.nice.org accessed January 2007).

There is no doubt that surgery has a place in the current management of obesity. A recent study showed that after obesity surgery, patients experienced complete resolution or improvement of their co-morbid conditions, including diabetes, hypertension, hyperlipidaemia and obstructive sleep apnoea.[13]

Weight loss as a consequence of surgery may have a positive impact on a person unable to work because of either gross excess weight or the co-morbidities associated with it. But it is neither readily available in the UK nor, for some patients, does it prevent future weight gain. For some individuals, a graph of weight against time has a depressing upward trend but, having lost significant weight, they will still have years of improved lipids, lower blood pressure and reduced health risks. One important consequence of bariatric surgery, however, is the need in a significant number of patients for further surgery by plastic surgeons to remove the large amounts of skin and loose tissue which result from weight loss. This may be needed on the arms and on the abdomen. Patients need to be aware of the possibility of this and the fact that it will not be performed until their weight has stabilised and further weight loss becomes unlikely.

WHAT DOES THE FUTURE HOLD?

The field of therapeutics for obesity is currently very active. Researchers are looking at chemical hormones released when we eat and their influence on appetite and sensations of fullness, and on chemicals in the brain which drive us to start and to stop eating.

Innovation is taking place in the field of surgery, with implantable gastric stimulation. This minimally invasive surgical approach is not in widespread use and its place in treatment needs to be better defined. The technique involves placing an implanted electric pulse generator in the abdomen. A wire connects the small battery-operated stimulator to the stomach wall. A small electric current is delivered to the lesser curve of the stomach wall, causing it to relax and expand, signalling a feeling of fullness and satiety to the brain. There have been over 600 implants inserted worldwide and, with the correct surgical training, the technique has few side-effects as it is a minimally invasive laparoscopic procedure performed as an outpatient service.[14]

KEY POINTS

- ∞ The mainstay of management of obesity is to lose small amounts of weight on a weekly basis through diet and physical activity.
- ∞ Medication may be needed for high BMIs in addition to the above.
- ∞ For obese people and people with co-morbidities, surgery can be an option but its availability is limited.

REFERENCES

1 Department of Health. *Choosing a Better Diet: a food and health action plan.* London; March 2005.

2 Kosasek *et al. Nutrition Today* 1991; November–December: 25–31.

3 Department of Health. *Choosing Activity: a physical action plan.* London; 2005

4 Department for Transport. *National Travel Survey 1999–2001: update.* London: Department for Transport; 2001.

5 National Institute for Clinical Excellence. *Guidance on the use of orlistat for the treatment of obesity in adults.* Technology Appraisal Guidance No. 22. London: NICE; 2001.

6 National Institute for Clinical Excellence. *Guidance on the use of sibutramine for the treatment of obesity in adults.* Technology Appraisal Guidance No. 31. London: NICE; 2001.

7 Nashund I, Agten G. Is obesity surgery worthwhile? *Obes Surg.* 1999; **9**: 36.

8 Kral JG. Obesity. In: Lubin MF *et al.* editors. *Medical Management of the Surgical Patient.* 3rd ed. Philadelphia, US: Lippincott; 1995.

9 Belachew H, Legnand M, Vincent V *et al.* Laparoscopic adjustable gastric banding. *Werla Gunnel Surgery.* 1998; **22**: 955–63.

10 Scottish Intercollegiate Guidelines Network. *Obesity in Scotland: integrating prevention with weight management.* Scottish Intercollegiate Guidelines Network; 1996.

11 Mason EE, Tang S, Requiat KE *et al.* Decade of change in obesity surgery. *Obes Surg.* 1997; **7**: 189–97.

12 National Institute for Clinical Excellence. *Guidance on the use of surgery to aid weight reduction for people with morbid obesity.* Technology Appraisal Guidance No. 46. London: NICE; 2002.

13 Buchwald H, Avidor Y, Braunwald E *et al.* Bariatric surgery: a systematic review and meta analysis. *JAMA* 2004 October; **292** (14): 1728.

14 Rankin D. The IGS: a new surgical approach. *Obesity News Review – Journal of the National Obesity Forum.* issue 10; February 2005.

CHAPTER 7

The workplace setting: improving nutrition and promoting physical activity

> 'The only important things in life are food, sex and work.'
>
> SIGMUND FREUD

Having in previous chapters considered the background and scale of the obesity problem, the medical issues and implications for the workplace, and reviewed the current options for clinical management, this chapter deals with the workplace and provides examples of what can be done to make it healthier, both for people who are overweight and obese already and for those yet to carry excessive weight. The perspective is deliberately global, as many key messages can be found in schemes set up for migrant workers and people with poor nutritional status as well as in initiatives to improve workplaces and make them better and thus more productive.

Large-scale interventions and screening programmes for obesity at workplaces have been well established across the world.[1] Some examples are:

- the national healthcare system in Cuba, which aims to prevent nutrition-related non-communicable diseases by taking out information and advice into workplaces
- work sites in Chile, which are used for screening for risk factors for non-communicable diseases
- a large-scale, multi-site intervention in India which has addressed exercise, changes in cafeteria menus and counselling on the nutrition of the family
- regular health screenings, health and nutrition education and counselling for workers in South Korea and
- the promotion of physical activity through work in Thailand as part of the National Plan with regional implementation.

Until recently, in the UK, the workplace was not truly recognised as presenting an opportunity to improve the health of the working population. The first sign of a change in emphasis was the World Health Organisation's Report 'WHO global strategy on diet, physical activity and health', published in 2004,[2] which mentioned the importance of fruit and vegetables in the workplace. A further sign of change can also be seen in the UK Government's White Paper 'Choosing health', which specifically mentions the benefits of the use of the workplace as a site for health promotion.[3]

Workplaces are attractive as possible sites to deliver health messages for several reasons.

1   The population is essentially 'captive' so potentially large numbers of people can be targeted at any one time, making programmes efficient.

2   The working population contains individuals who do not visit their doctors or primary care centres frequently and so may not be picking up health messages or accessing services.

3   Some employers have a positive commitment to employee health and will fund programmes beyond that which local services can usually provide.

4   Opportunities for follow-up and for assessing the effectiveness of interventions are greater than in community studies.

5   It is much easier to manipulate the working environment than it is the home or social environment, so positive action can be taken at the workplace both to help people maintain their current weight and to help others lose weight.

6   Many workplaces have access to specialist occupational health physicians and nurses who are some of the few health professionals who have an understanding of the whole business environment and its interactions with health from all angles (effects of health on work, work on health, rehabilitation and health promotion).

7   There is increasing interest in companies about the links between overweight and obesity and sickness absence, ill-health retirement and 'presenteeism' – the concept of attendance at work but reduced productivity due to chronic ill-health, which is gaining credibility in the US.

The workplace offers huge opportunities both to prevent weight gain and to aid weight loss through interventions in nutrition and physical activity, but why should businesses bother to do anything? The argument for action can be divided into reasons relating to health, safety, corporate social responsibility, moral and ethical stances.

HEALTH ISSUES

The co-morbidities associated with obesity, and the frequency of the condition, mean that there are strong economic reasons for taking action. Overweight and obese people are reported to have increased short- and long-term sickness absence rates when compared to people of normal weight. This translates into both direct costs (of sick pay) and indirect costs (of agency cover, training others to take on roles etc.). Because of the increased risk of cardiovascular disease and diabetes, there is an increased risk of early retirement on health grounds, with early payment of pensions and the costs of ill-health retirement. Probably few businesses could truly evaluate the cost of obesity to the business because, in many instances, it is the complications of the condition which appear on doctor's letters and medical reports and on sickness certificates.

SAFETY ISSUES

The increased risk of occupational accidents in obese people is a powerful argument for all employers, no matter the size of the company or the industrial sector in which they operate, to consider the impact of obesity on their business. Similarly the increased risk of road traffic accidents affects particularly those businesses with large sales forces or involved in delivery of goods, but all employers have employees who drive to work and who take sick leave if they are involved in road traffic accidents.

The use of all types of personal protective equipment is fundamental to the protection of workers across many industries and in the prevention of transmission of infection, particularly in healthcare. Body shape changes dramatically as weight accumulates and the ergonomic fit of personal protective equipment can be compromised. Purchasing custom-made items is both time-consuming and expensive but may be the only way for a particularly large employee to be adequately protected.

CORPORATE SOCIAL RESPONSIBILITY (CSR)

The CSR movement is based on the premise that an employer who is seen to contribute to the community and take responsibilities regarding environment, health and safety and waste management, is an employer whose business will benefit through easier recruitment and retention of staff and better appreciation of being a 'good' business, thus attracting more customers. Companies with CSR policies and activities are thought to be valued by employees who, in turn, are more productive. A CSR initiative by a food company to assist staff in making healthy nutritional choices and to provide opportunities for physical activity, may be seen as a responsible action by an organisation which cares about its products and how they are used. Similarly a car company may develop a CSR initiative to lay cycle paths and routes to show it is sensitive to the needs of both the environment and climate change and also to the health of its workers.

MORAL AND ETHICAL ASPECTS

Linked with CSR is the company who wishes to portray an image of a caring employer who morally believes in assisting in the welfare of staff. There is a strong history tradition of such approaches from companies such as Rowntree and Cadburys in the UK, whose founders provided high-quality housing and sports facilities for employees of their food factories.

Some companies and senior managers believe that business has far more responsibility towards staff than just what the law demands and that, by subsidising healthy options and activity opportunities, they are fulfilling a moral obligation as an employer that is a 'must do' rather than a 'might do'.

PREPARATION

Knowing the drivers that operate in various businesses is essential to the successful influencing of senior managers to make changes in the workplace. Thus a proposal to subsidise cycle purchase, to encourage cycle use to get to work and thus increase physical activity, may fit in with the company's green transport policy as well as being viewed as a perk by staff. All avenues need to be explored to facilitate and support health promotion initiatives, including the personal interests of those with influence.

Key ingredients to successful workplace interventions

The workplace is not the same as other settings for health promotion. Participation by businesses and individuals is entirely voluntary and these are not patients but workers. It should not be assumed that all employers will welcome such a pro- gramme without reservations. Most commonly there are concerns that, whatever is done, it will take people away from their jobs and cause *disruption* to the basic purpose of their being there – to work! Less commonly there are concerns about *equity of access* across the business – some programmes operate only at head offices when it is the staff working in operational roles in the field who lead a more sedentary lifestyle and so may need more support. *Cost* may be an issue for the delivery of the programme and for the materials used. Finally, *failure to provide feedback* to management on the uptake and success of the programme reduces the likelihood of future proposals being accepted.

The key ingredients to a successful workplace weight management programme include:

- research to identify key business drivers and why the particular business may be willing to sign up to a weight management programme

- buy-in and support from key figures in the business and in each workplace. This may be the chief executive, a director or Human Resource professional
- communication with existing healthcare professionals working for the business. This is a basic courtesy and essential for success. Some businesses operate as autonomous business units and may contract in an occupational service but seek to undertake a health promotion programme with a different provider. Communication between the two is essential to ensure understanding of the goals and how the two services interact
- support from unions or worker representatives
- careful consideration of any fitness-for-work issues. Some medical conditions associated with obesity may have implications for an individual's ability to drive, mount an emergency response or be in a safety critical role. Any implications for fitness for work need to be evaluated *prior* to any screening programme being established, as there may be significant industrial relations implications
- any initiative needs clear consistent leadership throughout the life of the project
- if a health promotion programme or initiative can be integrated into other initiatives, such as green transport policies, it has a better chance of being sustainable and continuing after the inevitable reduction of enthusiasm following its start
- initiatives which rely on just one individual driving them forward are in danger of collapse if that individual leaves the organisation, is ill or is relocated to a different job. A team approach is more effective in terms of ideas, lessons learnt and sustainability
- a clear idea, in advance of any action, to decide what is to be done, who needs to do it, over what time course and what it is hoped will be achieved. A similarly clear idea of the budget for the whole project, how it will be spent and when, is also fundamental
- finally, an evaluation plan needs to be drawn up before initiation. What are the measures of success? What are the timelines for report-backs to be made? What will be the form and content of the report-back to the business? and most important . . . What sort of information can be fed back which will influence continuation of the initiative, further funding or another health promotion activity?

'SELLING' THE CONCEPT OF WEIGHT MANAGEMENT

Most people are interested in weight, either in relation to themselves, their families or children. Many staff will be current or historical dieters, so it's likely that there will be enthusiasm for weight management from a significant proportion of any working population. Gauging how much enthusiasm and likely uptake of any initiative is needed to manage the budget and use resources appropriately.

The key message in 'selling' the concept of a programme or initiative to business is that a lot can be achieved even with no budget, though greater options clearly exist with a small or larger budget.

WHAT CAN BE ACHIEVED WITH NO BUDGET

Initiatives to improve nutrition

- Look at food labelling – work with caterers to label healthy options. Some companies use a traffic light system for fat, sugar and salt content. Labelling meals with 'points' to help people following the Weight Watchers plan can also help workers make informed choices.
- Work with sandwich vendors to offer healthier options and include fruit.
- Encourage caterers to organise sampling sessions and serve fruit smoothies and low-fat, low-salt dishes.
- Work with vending machine suppliers to place water and healthy fruit drinks in prominent positions in machines and move the high-sugar drinks out of eye line.

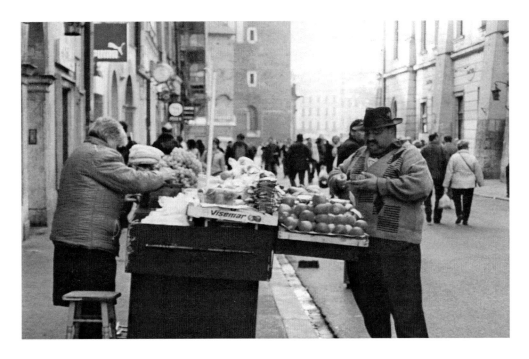

Fresh fruit and vegetables bought locally. © N Williams.

- Encourage the use of local vendors serving fresh fruit and vegetables outside work premises or bring fruit and vegetable vendors into the workplace.
- Remove salt from the tables in the canteen/restaurant and instead make it available on request.
- Download free healthy eating advice from organisations such as the Food Standards Agency (*see* Chapter 11, Further resources) and display it in the canteen.
- Place healthy eating messages and promote any initiative with messages in pay packets and on company notice boards. A campaign type of approach could be used – e.g. Low Fat Week – which provides information on notice boards, highlights options in the canteen and runs simple quizzes to test knowledge and educate. The prize could be a healthy meal or basket of fruit.

CASE STUDY 7.1

Merthyr Tydfil Housing Association employees 36 staff across three sites in Wales. It provides homes and services for people on low incomes.
  The company:
- set up themed days for promoting health, including healthy eating, and used designated notice boards for health promotion topics
- arranged discounted fitness club membership and evaluated the success of the scheme by gym attendance, which increased.

Initiatives to promote physical activity

- Have a 'no email' day. Companies who declare one day email free have found that staff walk over to colleagues more.
- Encourage greater use of stairs. Many stairs look as if they should only be used in emergencies and not as routine walkways. Look at the stairs around the company and suggest ways of increasing their usage, e.g. by setting up picture galleries on the landings and inviting employees to display their children's art work. Make sure the safety officer is involved in any ideas and that they check that the stairs are well lit and hazard free.
- Alternatively, place data graphs with information concerning production, complaints and compliments on landings.
- Publicise local sports facilities on company intranet sites and notice boards.
- Participate in schemes to encourage cycle use by negotiating discounts with local retailers and advertising them on company intranet sites and notice boards.
- Use a pedometer to mark up walking trails around the workplace and work out the number of steps between departments. Encourage people to increase the number of steps they take per day and to choose longer routes between office buildings and departments. Work out the additional steps which would

be taken per day if someone parked their car at the furthermost point of the car park compared to parking as near as possible to the entrance.

CASE STUDY 7.2

St George's University, Grenada, West Indies, is visited by vendors on a daily basis. The vendors sell fresh fruit and vegetables to students and staff as they are waiting for buses.

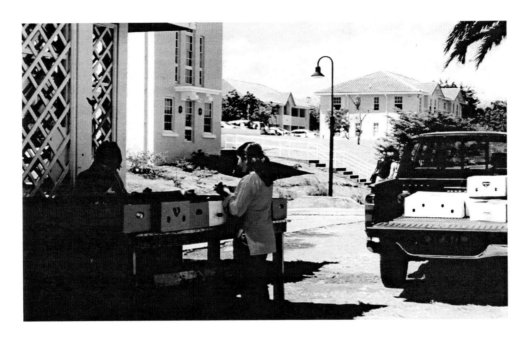

Onsite fruit and vegetable sales on campus. St George's University, Grenada, West Indies.
© N Williams.

CASE STUDY 7.3

Knock Travel, a Belfast-based provider of leisure and business travel, took several actions for healthy eating (outlined in Case study 7.5) and these were complemented by a Stepometer challenge over one week to see who could take the most steps. Staff also formed a walking group in the lunch time.

Doreen McKenzie, proprietor, said 'these initiatives truly have been of benefit to us as a company, as well as to our staff and customers. The results increase the bottom line, so I can heartily recommend any employer to look at the issues even from a purely commercial perspective.' (Reported in *Health, Work and Well Being – caring for our future. Case studies*. DWP: London; 2006.)

CASE STUDY 7.4

Heart of Birmingham (HOB) has a green transport plan which aims to encourage staff to cycle to work and use means other than their cars, so as to reduce environmental damage and to ease pressure on parking at the NHS Trust. To complement the plan, the Trust worked with Halfords, a national company selling bicycles, to provide a Bikes4Work scheme. Details of the scheme were placed on the Trust's intranet site and road shows took place at the two hospital sites at which workers could see and try various bicycles. Those interested then applied for a voucher for between £100 and £1000 (about $180 US) to purchase a bicycle and accessories at any of the company's stores. The voucher value was deducted through their salary over an 18-month period but also gave tax and national insurance relief on the payments made. This meant that workers received a 30% discount on their purchase.

WHAT CAN BE ACHIEVED WITH A SMALL BUDGET

Initiatives to improve nutrition

- Subsidies on the healthy options in canteens/restaurants and vending machines. Caterers and vending machine operators know how many portions of various foods, drinks and snacks sell, so it should be possible to estimate costs accurately in advance of any change in pricing.
- Invite the local NHS dietician or local health promotion team at the primary care trust to provide a presentation or literature on how to read food labels.
- Offer smoothies (low-fat) at meetings along with tea and coffee.
- Remove sweets from reception areas and replace with fruit and nuts.

CASE STUDY 7.5

Knock Travel, a Belfast-based provider of leisure and business travel, undertook several initiatives to improve the health and well-being of its staff. The company:
- installed two kitchens and provided microwave ovens so staff could have a hot meal and bring in food from home to eat
- arranged fruit weeks (provision of different fruits for a week, showing healthier benefits) and held a similar vegetable week
- held a 'smoothie' day
- arranged for a dietician to come to talk and provide information on healthy eating.

Initiatives to promote physical activity

- Set up a cycle pool and allow staff to borrow bikes to cycle between sites and to and from work.

- Operate a subsidised pedometer purchase scheme.
- Subsidise swimming and gym use by staff.
- Offer prizes for individuals or teams for participation in physical activity. Offer a cash donation to a local charity based on staff weight loss or physical activity. Sponsoring staff in charity walks or runs can also be undertaken and it gains publicity for the company in local newspapers.
- Provide information and promote the use of cycles in addition to public transport. Lobby local councils and transport services for better cycle parks, such as those provided in Oxford, where reliable secure cycling ranks and facilities have helped to reduce city traffic and promote healthy physical activity – and not only among its student population.

CASE STUDY 7.6

A local council in southern England established a bike pool to allow staff to borrow a bike to cycle to work. One man in his 40s with a sedentary job joined the scheme and found that, not only was he fitter after just six weeks and able to complete his home-to-work journey much quicker, but he also felt his general level of alertness increased.

(Reported in *The Sunday Times*, 13 November 2005.)

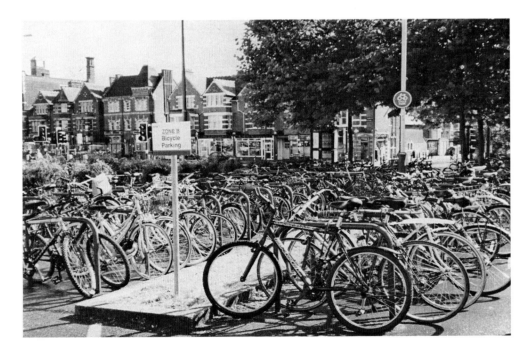

Cycle park at Oxford Interchange, UK. © N Williams.

CASE STUDY 7.7

Manchester Airport has over 2000 employees and many service partners. It actively encourages cycling by laying out cycle paths round the airport and by having an onsite repair and maintenance cycle centre.

CASE STUDY 7.8

A walking initiative at GlaxoSmithKline (GSK) used pedometers as a means to promote physical activity in the workplace. The project developed as a result of a health risk appraisal which identified low levels of physical activity among employees. This was believed to be because many people were unaware of the level of physical activity required to offer health gains. Consequently, a stock of pedometers was purchased from the Countryside Agency for the launch of the programme. Roadshow-style events were held across GSK sites, in partnership with physical activity specialists. These served to increase awareness of pedometers and gave employees the chance to see and experience how pedometers work. Interest was maintained by the development of a website which included an online purchasing form and support materials for the programme which staff could access. This proved very popular, as over 1200 pedometers were bought across 20 GSK sites. (Reproduced with permission of GSK.)

CASE STUDY 7.9

Merseyside Travelwise specialises in working in partnership with businesses and organisations in order to produce travel plans promoting efficient and healthy travel. The Travelwise Merseyside campaign promotes the benefits of walking, cycling and public transport, including the positive health benefits. It is centred around working with businesses and organisations to develop travel plans and help provide sustainable alternatives to make it easier for people to use an active way of travelling to work to improve their health.

Practical measures are developed in association with employees and employers, with the aim of reducing car dependency and encouraging the use of sustainable modes of transport.

These include:

- improving pedestrian access for employees and visitors by improving signage and access points
- promoting the health benefits of walking
- encouraging walking to and from site meetings
- organising walking clubs for lunchtimes and after work
- making sure that access points for pedestrians are safe, well lit and convenient for local transport routes
- providing lockers, changing facilities and showers

- providing 'pool bikes'
- offering financial incentives for active travel
- providing travel maps and information on local cycle routes.
  (Reproduced with permission from Merseyside Travelwise, www.LetsTravelWise.org.uk)

WHAT CAN BE ACHIEVED WITH A LARGER BUDGET

Initiatives to improve nutrition

- Provide fruit free to staff on a daily basis.
- Make healthy options free of charge.
- Replace buffet lunches and use portion-controlled individual portions of low-fat, low-salt food for all meetings and conferences.
- Set up a weight management programme involving individualised assessment of diet and provide specific advice. Arrange follow-up and provide supporting materials and information help lines.
- Provide water, plain and flavoured with fruit, free of charge during work.

Initiatives to promote physical activity

- Provide a gym at work or fund membership of one of the national gym chains.
- Provide free Pilates, yoga and exercise classes in lunch times and after work.
- Provide rewards for those participating in exercise, e.g. time off to participate during work hours.
- Set up and sponsor a company football, netball, hockey or cricket team.
- Arrange for personalised fitness assessment for staff with plans for improvement and increased activity.

CASE STUDY 7.10

The Dole Food Company Inc. California is the world's largest producer of fresh fruit, vegetables and packaged goods. It has an educational outreach programme aimed at communities and school children and has been proactive in workplace initiatives to promote healthy eating. Key features of its action include free morning and afternoon fruit and vegetable breaks, onsite weekly farmers markets, an onsite dietician, bi-weekly newsletters on fitness and health and access to physical activities. The company awards 'Dole dollars' for employees who participate in its Dole Employee Wellness (DEW) programme, which can be redeemed for gift certificates. On any given day 75% of employees use the canteen and they are offered a range of healthy options, including vegetarian and vegan options. Food is heavily subsidised, with breakfasts costing $3 (about £2.10) and a daily Dole Special lunch for $4.25 (about £3). There is no beef, pork, cream, whole milk or sugary drinks and non-healthy options on sale. It represents an unusual 'all or nothing' approach. Dole has conducted a financial evaluation of the cost of setting up the initiative ($100 000 in the first year) and is working on an evaluation of the benefits. From a public relations perspective, Dole has received a lot of very favourable publicity in newspapers and industry trade journals and feels the scheme has benefited worker recruitment and retention as well as assisting some employees to lose weight – 'sometimes without trying'. It has also received favourable publicity in trade press and newspapers and has been praised by US politicians.

(Case study edited and reproduced with permission from *Food at Work* by Christopher Wanjek. ILO Geneva. Copyright 2005 International Labour Organization.)

CASE STUDY 7.11

A Scottish university developed a comprehensive physical activity policy and facilities, allowed time and provided support for exercise throughout the day. It provided a covered and secure cycle area, showers, gym facilities and arranged walking and jogging groups and fitness classes at lunch time. The university plans to reward staff who participate with an hour of exercise which can be taken from their working day. It has also encouraged more walking by placing walking signs around the campus.

CASE STUDY 7.12

The Canadian company Telus (formerly BC Telecom) developed a wellness programme in 1977. It reported fitness programme members were 28% less absent from work when compared to the general employee population: 94% were more productive and 86% reported that their physical activity helped them to manage stress better.[4] Both occupational health and fitness trainers provided information on weight management, and nutrition counselling for employees and their families was provided by a certified dietician. Telus received the 1999 Healthy Workplace Award from the National Quality Institute for its commitment to the health of its employees.

CASE STUDY 7.13

Fruitions Limited is a health promotion/lifestyle company which provides weight management programmes for businesses of all sizes. At one client in the West Midlands, they had several individual successes which illustrate the impact such a programme can have.

Example 7.13a

Before: Mr X was a 54-year-old type 2 diabetic, hypertensive and clinically obese, with a BMI of over 39 kg/m². He did not undertake any form of exercise and could not comfortably walk half a mile. He was struggling to move around at work in the afternoons.

After: Mr X had regular sessions with the lifestyle manager and by 18 months had lost three stone (19 kg) and 10% of his body fat. His BMI reduced to just over 33. He had started to walk regularly at lunch time and had inspired several colleagues to join him. Having walked up Mount Snowdon and Mount Ben Nevis, he had set himself the goal of walking in the Alps. He no longer felt that he struggled at work in the afternoons.

Example 7.13b

Before: Mr Y was a 51-year-old maintenance manager. He was required to climb ladders and fit into confined spaces, however, he was finding this difficult. He was clinically obese (BMI over 44 kg/m²) and was severely restricted in his agility and ability to get around. He had no co-morbidities but, away from work, he avoided playing tennis with his daughter, as he knew he was not fit enough.

After: At 12 months Mr Y had lost 4 stone (25.5 kg) and his BMI had reduced to 38. He was able to tackle more tasks at work and felt more confident in undertaking the tasks required of him. He also felt he had more energy during the day. His family had benefited from his healthy-eating regime, which had now become the norm.

(Case studies reproduced with the permission of Fruitions Limited.)

KEY POINTS

What employers can do:

∞ reflect on the impact of obesity on business and customer relationships

∞ identify what resources, facilities and schemes are available locally to encourage increased physical activity and better nutrition and how they can be accessed

∞ review food available in the workplace – in reception, the canteen/restaurant and snack bars, and in vending machines and factory shops

∞ encourage exercise by investigating tax breaks for cycles, providing bike racks and security facilities, and contact national chains of gyms and health clubs to negotiate membership reductions for staff

∞ provide information on healthy eating and on food labelling

∞ support staff in their efforts to lose weight through sponsorship and team competitions

∞ explore if a weight management initiative might help local projects and improve relationships between the business and the local community

∞   signpost employees to web and self-help resources to help them lose weight.

REFERENCES

1 Doak C. Large-scale interventions and programmes addressing nutrition-related chronic diseases and obesity: examples from 14 counties. *Public Health Nutr.* 2002; **5** (1A): 275–7.

2 World Health Organisation. *Global strategy on diet, physical activity and health.* Annex of WHO Assembly Resolution WHA57.17, paragraph 62. Geneva; 22 May 2004.

3 Department of Health. *Choosing Health: making healthy choices easier.* 2004. www. dh.gov.uk (accessed February 2005).

4 Gault M. Shedding the burden. *Canadian Occupational Safety* 2000; **38** (3): 23–6.

CHAPTER 8

Workplace design: improving nutrition and promoting physical activity

> 'You are old', said the youth, 'As I mentioned before,
> And have grown most uncommonly fat.
> Yet you turned a back-somersault in at the door –
> Pray what was the reason of that?'

LEWIS CARROLL 'ALICE'S ADVENTURES UNDER GROUND'

As a specialty, occupational medicine aims to prevent ill-health caused by work and to improve the health of the working population. It is now well recognised that work, if properly organised, can improve health, particularly mental health, and with our aging population in the Western world, more and more people are needed to remain in employment to fund the health and social care that our elderly population expect.

Obesity and other conditions such as smoking cause far more deaths world-wide than occupational accidents and occupational cancers, but they are multi-factorial in origin and owe a lot to behaviour learnt and practised outside the workplace.

That said, the workplace offers an unrivalled opportunity to apply the principles of prevention of occupational ill-health to these common public health issues.

Classically, risk reduction as applied to agents such as chemicals, involves a hierarchy of measures.
- Firstly, aim to eliminate the hazardous agent.
- If it cannot be eliminated, then substitute it for something safer.
- Put controls in place to prevent exposure.
- Check that the controls are working.

- Provide health surveillance to check for any residual risk.
- Provide information, instruction and training.

To manage obesity in the workplace, it is tempting just to look at putting in place better nutritional information and encouraging exercise, but a similar set of hierarchical measures could be applied.

- Eliminate poor food and sedentary work design. (*See* Case studies 8.1, 8.2 and 8.3.)
- Substitute with low-fat, low-salt healthy foods and provide for physical activity. (*See* Case study 8.4.)
- Check these foods and drinks are attractive and accessed (checking controls). (*See* Case study 8.5.)
- Provide health promotion so people learn about food and activity and can make healthy choices for themselves. (*See* Case study 8.6.)
- Provide information, instruction and training in how to select food, portion size, and benefits of various types of activity. (*See* Case study 8.7.)

CASE STUDY 8.1

The Radisson SAS Hotel, Edinburgh, is part of an international chain of hotels. On request, they produced special healthy options menus and food for a conference of health specialists in December 2005. Menus were agreed in advance with the conference organisers and aimed to meet various dietary needs and food preferences with a varied choice of low-fat food options with lots of fruit and vegetables.

In addition to tea and coffee, the hotel provided still and sparkling water and strawberry and banana smoothies at break times in the morning and afternoon. The smoothies were particularly popular as an alternative to caffeine-containing drinks.

For lunch on Day 1, the menu consisted of:
Chicken on skewers
Warm pitta bread with hummus
Breadsticks
Foccacia bread with tuna and tomato
Guacamole and salsa wraps
Ham and mustard sandwiches (brown bread)

For dinner on Day 1, the menu was:
Platter of seasonal fruits and raspberry syrup
Roast supreme of salmon with a white wine and chive sauce and selection of
  steamed vegetables
Individual orange cheesecake with berry coulis.

For lunch on Day 2, the menu was:
    Salmon on skewers
    Beef and bean casserole
    Vegetables fricassee
    Prawn salad
    Spinach tortilla with tomato and coriander salad
    Sweet pepper and courgette sandwich
    Selection of fresh fruit and yoghurts

The high standard of appearance, quality and taste of the food was commented on by delegates throughout the conference.
    (Reproduced with kind permission of the Radisson Hotel, Edinburgh.)

CASE STUDY 8.2

Recent reports about innovations in the Mayo Clinic in the US have described how walking on a treadmill at about 1 mph whilst answering emails can burn as many as 1000 calories per day. The researchers have designed and developed a treadmill workstation which removes the sedentary nature of desk jobs. The computer is located at chest height on a small platform with a conventional keyboard. This is part of their 'Office of the Future' initiative, which includes setting up two-lane walking tracks so meetings are held on the go. More information is available from their website, www.mayoclinic.org/news2005-rst/2836.html

CASE STUDY 8.3

A large manufacturing company in the UK has abolished seated meetings. All meetings now take place standing up. Consequently they tend to be shorter and more focused, with a higher level of physical activity recorded on pedometers during the working day.

CASE STUDY 8.4

San Pedro Disenos is a small textile company in Guatemala, South America. Its workers are low wage earners, many of whom are poorly educated. Wages are based on productivity but an occupational health and safety programme found that they often missed breakfast and many did not have suitable lunch. There was little understanding about nutrition and what was known was learnt from the media and television and was often incorrect. The company brought in an hour-long lunch break and provided cooking facilities and a dining area. Free bread was provided and free coffee during breaks. The company subsidised the cost of breakfast and lunch by about $2 US per meal and found that, since the introduction of the programme, workers are more productive, morale is higher and absenteeism has fallen along with medical costs.

(Reproduced with kind permission from *Food at Work* by C Wanjek. ILO Geneva. Copyright 2005 International Labour Organization.)

CASE STUDY 8.5

A Danish workplace initiative, Firmafrugt, aimed to increase fruit and vegetable consumption and had several components, including one focused on catering. Five demonstration canteens worked with increasing amounts of fruit and vegetables available for purchase. Personnel and management and the catering team worked closely with the project personnel. Intake was measured by weighing fruit and vegetables served minus baseline, during the intervention and at one year follow-up. Significant increases in fruit and vegetable intake were shown at all five demonstration sites, on average 70 g per day per customer, bringing the intake to an average 95 g per day per customer.

Businesses have latched onto the initiative and participation increased from 623 workplaces in 2001 to nearly 5000 in 2003 and over 9200 in 2004. This latter figure represents 9% of the Danish workforce. The fruit is simple and is displayed in baskets with disposable towels available. There is usually one piece of fruit available per worker per shift. Workers consider that Firmafrugt is a sign that the company cares about them.

(Edited and reproduced with permission from *Food at Work* by C Wanjek ILO. Copyright 2005 International Labour Organization.)

CASE STUDY 8.6

General Electric Company (GEC) has a Health by Numbers programme which asks employees to achieve four personal numbers: 0 for smoking, 5 for fruit and vegetable servings per day, 10 000 for steps taken per day, and 25 for their BMI target. Employees manage their personal health through web-based information sources and programmes to help them achieve each behavioural goal. GEC's programme won them a 'Best Employer for Healthy Lifestyles Award' from the National Business Group on Health, a non-profit organisation devoted exclusively to representing large employers' perspective on national health policy issues and providing practical solutions to its members' most important health care problems. Best Employer for Healthy Lifestyles Awards recognise and reward companies across the US that apply creative solutions to improving the health of employees.

(Reproduced with kind permission from the National Business Group on Health; 2006.)

CASE STUDY 8.7

Selecta is a UK catering company and provider of vending machine contents. It has started to educate users as to the nutritional contents of the machines by placing brightly covered stickers and information on fat, sugar and calories on the machines themselves so that employees can make healthier choices.

CASE STUDY 8.8

The owner of a US company employing 200 people, having forced his employees to give up smoking or give up their job, has now adopted a hardline attitude towards excess weight. Employees are given $35 (about £19) per month as an incentive to go to the gym and another $65 (about £35) if they meet fitness targets set for them. The results of the weight incentive are pending but his approach to smoking led to 20 workers giving up. When interviewed he is reported as saying 'I'm not controlling their lives. They have a choice if they want to work here.'[1]

KEY MESSAGES FOR WORKPLACE PROGRAMMES

Initiatives need to:
- make it easy to make healthy choices
- make it harder to make unhealthy choices
- offer a range of options – one size does not fit all
- provide rewards (not necessarily financial) for participation and success
- celebrate success internally and externally
- ensure that evaluation is a fundamental part of any initiative.

KEY POINTS

- ∞ The workplace can be the setting for a range of initiatives to promote healthier eating and greater physical activity.

- ∞ Budgets do not have to be large but creative thinking can help develop interesting and innovative schemes.

- ∞ One feature of health-based initiatives is their focus on employees – the initiatives are often seen as a sign that the employer values their employees and cares about their well-being. Benefits, difficult to measure as they are, may therefore extend beyond improved health for the employees, to improved health of the business.

REFERENCE

1 Litterick, D. Fat staff ordered to shape up or ship out. *Telegraph*. 28 January 2005.

Health promotion: work task and workplace redesign and population approaches

> 'To the people, food is heaven.'

<small>CHINESE PROVERB</small>

The field of health promotion is so vast that it really deserves a book to itself but in this chapter I hope to condense some of the words of wisdom and much of the philosophy and practice in the field. Much of the literature is not relevant to the workplace and shows little insight into the differences in the workplace setting compared to primary care and communities, but many of the basic principles are the same.

PREPARATION

Before embarking on any programme it is crucial to start with the most basic information, such as:

- financial resources available
- human resources available
- the key drivers for the workplace and the workers
- important limiting factors
- complementary company initiatives
- the need for leadership and commitment
- the type of evaluation needed and what success looks like.

What is needed in broad terms is:

- a *strategy* informed by data (e.g. on sickness absence rates, numbers for ill-health retirement, results of health screening programmes, employee satisfaction and valuation questionnaires)

▌ a *plan* on what to do and over what time course. Is this a campaign (either standing alone or linking with a national campaign, e.g. Men's Health Week) or is it an ongoing initiative integrated into wellness or occupational health programmes? There may be certain times of the year when a campaign is more appealing – e.g. for a weight reduction campaign, New Year resolutions to lose weight after the holidays may increase participation. 'Get fit for summer' may support a physical activity programme.

Key points in the year are:
▐ **January** – New Year resolutions (e.g. 'Shed those Christmas calories')
▐ **May–June** – pre-holiday campaigns (e.g. 'Get fit for summer')
▐ **September–October** – post-holiday campaigns (e.g. 'Prepare for Christmas – lose a few pounds now and save yourself the New Year resolution!'

But encouraging staff to keep weight off all year is more likely to bring about significant changes. These additional initiatives can support an underlying supportive programme such as that used at Pitney Bowes (*see* Case study 9.1).

▌ a *communications strategy and plan.* How will employees be made aware of the initiative? How can they sign up? What communication messages need to be believed to encourage uptake and participation and make it clear 'what's in it for them'?
▌ an *action plan* describing exactly what the initiative is. Is it directed at improving nutrition, increasing physical activity, managing obesity? Is it aimed at influencing everyone or a target population? Does it involve choice or are unhealthy options and negative behaviours to be removed?
▌ an *evaluation plan.* What evaluation will be carried out and at what milestones? Will it be possible to record participation rates, changes in health/risk factors in individuals, or employee feedback on the value of the scheme to them and their families?
▌ clarity about *results* and their *communication.* What results will be produced and how will these be communicated to management, unions, worker representatives and staff?
▌ an understanding of what *publicity* will be generated about the initiative. Will there be participation in award schemes and articles submitted to the trade and healthcare press?

CASE STUDY 9.1

Pitney Bowes is a large, US-based worldwide organisation which recently won one of the Best Employers for Healthy Lifestyles Awards organised by the National Business Group on Health, a non profit organisation devoted exclusively to representing large employers' perspective on national health policy issues and providing practical solutions to its members' most important health care problems. Best Employer for Healthy Lifestyles Awards recognise and reward companies across the US that apply creative solutions to improving the health of employees.

The award recognised Pitney Bowes' achievements in developing a strategy using multiple channels of communication to answer 'What's in it for me?', and in increasing physical activity through the provision of walking paths, gym discounts and pedometers. The company also provided health risk assessments, lifestyle coaching and nutritional counselling for staff and evaluated the project, collecting data on participation rates and changes in health risks (reduced blood pressure, cholesterol etc.), as well as calculating the costs and effect on health claims.

The programme was called 'Maintain Don't Gain' and was designed to prevent cyclical holiday weight gain by asking staff to follow eight basic nutritional and health tips and by ensuring healthy labelled food was available in its canteens. The programme was run over just eight weeks, with the aim of stopping the 1–3 lb weight gain which an adult typically experiences in a year. In this initiative, success was measured by people maintaining their weight rather than gaining or losing pounds.

(Reproduced with kind permission of the National Business Group on Health.)

DECIDING WHETHER TO LOOK AT POPULATIONS OR INDIVIDUALS

In the workplace setting there are two fundamental approaches which could be applied to obesity management, either singly or in combination. Which to adopt depends on financial resources and on the available skill mix. Essentially, the options are either a campaign or a more consultation-based initiative.

The two basic approaches are either to concentrate on the whole working population and aim to maintain their weight – i.e. stopping people who are not yet overweight and obese from becoming so and raising awareness and encouraging people to lose weight with some support – or to adopt a targeted approach and seek out those who are already overweight and obese and help them to lose weight or at least not to gain further weight. Combinations of the two can also be undertaken – e.g. overall healthy eating awareness and canteen changes plus an offer to measure, weigh and monitor people who have BMIs over 27 kg/m^2.

From a public health perspective, the former is the more attractive as it is primary prevention of obesity rather than secondary prevention of the complications of the condition (heart attacks, strokes, diabetes and so forth). However, there is no doubt that it is the second group for whom relatively small changes in body weight can bring about large reductions in health risk profile. It is also the second group whose members are more likely to be having some difficulties in the workplace with mobility, fatigue or size issues.

A combination of the two approaches is ideal but can be more expensive. Another drawback of the combination approach is that it can make more difficult any evaluation of the success of the primary prevention approach, given the 'arms length' distance between the subjects and the programme initiator. For example, counting numbers of leaflets picked up does not relate to changes in behaviour. The person-focused approach, on the other hand, lends itself to easier evaluation with its hard outcomes such as kilograms of weight lost and numbers of people achieving significant health benefits through loss of 5–10% of their weight.

THE POPULATION APPROACH – WHAT COULD YOU DO?

With so many people in the working population now overweight or obese, population approaches are becoming increasingly effective as they reach large numbers of people and are neither labour intensive nor administratively intensive.

Depending on budget, commitment and company ethos, fundamental changes to workplace and work design can be undertaken. The benefits of not relying on employees to make choices and resist temptation is obvious – if you can change the underlying system, people don't have to make difficult choices and so weight maintenance and weight loss become easier and, I would argue, much more sustainable. Trying to integrate better nutrition and increase physical activity into daily work and presence at the workplace is likely to be far more effective than bolt-on healthy eating campaigns. The evidence for this comes from the health and safety field, where it has long been recognised that reliance on workers to use personal protective equipment (such as masks and overalls to protect themselves against chemicals) is much less effective than controlling the exposure to the agent at its source by putting in 'engineering controls'.

Applying the same philosophy to control calorie intake and increase energy expenditure is likely, in my view, to bring better and more sustainable results.

So what could be done? The following provides some examples of possible initiatives to address work tasks, the workplace environment and working populations. There will be many more, and not all are suited to each workplace, company or group of workers.

Types of common work environment: offices, shops and call centres

Few of us burn calories at work any more as most tasks are now performed seated at a computer, and with the advent of email, even walking over to colleagues has reduced. Hours spent sitting are a recipe for weight gain and this is anecdotally best seen on jobs such as call centre work, where workers may come from moderately active office jobs to a call centre where they sit and answer call after call, often without interruption except to visit the bathroom or get a drink. The result is weight gain and this can be significant especially with shift workers on the night shift, whose access to healthy food may be reduced.

Physical activity and the work task

In very sedentary jobs, interventions to improve physical activity aimed at the work task could include:

■ having an email free day once per week (encouraging walking around the office/centre)

■ making the meetings room a place for standing only (which also reduces the length of meetings)

■ providing tea points at locations where staff have to walk to them.

Physical activity and the workplace

In workplaces where very sedentary jobs take place, interventions to improve physical activity aimed at the workplace layout could include:

■ laying out a walking track around the workstations. Call centres are usually open plan, with teams working together. If not too cramped, laying a walking track and encouraging its use could also aid muscle relation and prevent back and upper limb pain

■ close siting of fresh water fountains/dispensers in the operational area. Encouraging use of water rather than soft drink also helps to prevent work-related voice disorders

■ marking out walking paths around the building and outside, including information on how many steps they take for completion. Displaying these routes on notice boards and on the company intranet is also useful. Similarly, relating the steps used to the minimum recommended steps (10 000 per day) and to the number of calories burnt and weight which can be lost just by increasing the number of steps daily (5000 steps = approx 200 calories).

Physical activity and the worker

For workers engaged in very sedentary tasks, interventions to improve physical activity aimed at workers themselves could include:

■ encouraging regular stretching and walking around the track, either alone or with a colleague. This also helps prevent back and upper limb pain from sustained static postures

■ encouraging the lunch break to be taken away from the desk and outside the building, preferably walking around a trail which has been marked out and for which the number of steps taken is roughly known

■ working out and advertising the number of steps from the office/call centre to local shops (where the office/centre is in a city location), then presenting this information in a positive light – e.g. 'Did you know that Telenorth to John Lewis is an amazing 3000 steps for a return journey? Make that journey and you are well on your way to the daily minimum.' And 'Did you know that two hours shopping on an afternoon can mean 2000 steps? Shopping can be good for your health!'

The aim is to increase walking in the course of the normal day. It is most likely to be successful if it encourages people to do more of what they enjoy doing anyway and so find that the increased activity is not a chore. Expecting people who have never thought about using a gym to suddenly go three or four times a week will be successful for only a small percentage of people. However, offering reduced gym membership to people who have already thought of using a gym may be the spur they need to take the first step.

There has to be a range of options to meet a range of likes and dislikes, social and financial circumstances and available time for different employees.

The same approach can be applied to improving nutrition in a call centre/office environment. Let's look at what it might mean.

Nutrition and the work task

In very sedentary jobs, interventions to improve nutrition aimed at the work task could include:

- ensuring an adequate lunch break to allow someone to leave the workstation and either buy healthy food locally or purchase it onsite
- providing water fountains/dispensers free of charge and allowing only water to be consumed at the workstation, with the aim of discouraging consumption of soft drinks.

Nutrition and the workplace

In workplaces where very sedentary jobs take place, interventions to improve nutrition aimed at the workplace layout could include:

- ensuring that vending facilities are loaded towards the healthy options being more plentiful, more visible and more attractively presented. Work with vending suppliers and consider subsidising healthy options (or even penalising unhealthy ones by increasing costs in order to remain cost neutral). Beware of removing all 'unhealthy' food as this is likely to lead to industrial relations issues, particularly with employees who do not have a weight problem but consume large quantities of unhealthy food. This is a matter of choice and persuasion rather than decree, and it is the hearts and minds of employees that we are seeking to influence.
- providing a small microwave area where employees can bring food in from home and hygienically prepare it.

Similar approaches can be applied to other occupational groups. One such example is given below.

Other types of worker: healthcare workers

Physical activity and the work task

In healthcare, interventions to improve physical activity aimed at the work task could include:

▌ providing cycles to get around hospital sites and having 'park and use' schemes.

Physical activity and the workplace

In workplaces where healthcare takes place, interventions to improve physical activity aimed at the workplace layout could include:

▌ reducing the number of parking spaces or increasing charges to encourage use of public transport and walking

▌ providing incentives for individuals living within two miles of a site to leave their cars behind

▌ seeking managerial agreement for staff to use out of hours the physiotherapy gym used by patients during the day.

Physical activity and the worker

For workers engaged in healthcare, interventions to improve physical activity aimed at workers themselves could include:

▌ advertising the number of steps need to walk down each long hospital corridor or from 'x ray to outpatients', 'accident and emergency to the canteen'

▌ declaring a 'lift-free' day when staff walk upstairs

▌ providing a basic set of scales in changing rooms – e.g. in theatre – to encourage weighing

▌ encouraging the setting-up of 'weight clubs' or 'weigh days' in different departments to highlight the need for weight to be monitored regularly.

Other types of worker: sales executives and business people, lawyers and accountants

Physical activity and the work task

In sales, business, law and accounts, interventions to improve physical activity aimed at the work task could include:

▌ arranging meetings outside of meal times

▌ avoiding business breakfasts and lunches where attention is diverted from portion size and volume of food consumed.

Physical activity and the workplace

In workplaces where sales, business, law and accountancy take place, interventions to improve physical activity aimed at the workplace layout could include:

▌ arranging accommodation only with hotel chains that offer room gyms, health facilities and healthy menus. Negotiate such additions as standard to rooms booked for each employee. Make it clear to travel agents and hotels that this is an important issue for your staff.

Physical activity and the worker

For workers engaged in sales, business, law and accountancy, interventions to improve physical activity aimed at workers themselves could include:

- dispelling the myth of the 'long hours' culture being a good thing for staff
- encouraging the use of exercise as a means of enhancing performance and rewarding staff who join gyms, take classes or use sporting facilities
- negotiating reduced rates at national gym chains for all staff
- ensuring that reduced-cost gym and exercise club membership is part of the rewards package on offer to staff and that it is extended to partners and family.

Other types of worker: truck drivers and delivery workers

Fixed workplaces are easier to impact on than remote, small, mobile or home-based workplaces. But for each occupational group, there are initiatives that can make healthy eating and increased physical activity a reality.

In the case of truck drivers and delivery workers who spend long periods on the road, with little opportunity to stop to eat at healthy venues, the fitting of a small fridge to stock salads, fruit and sandwiches could be a start. This group of workers is particularly vulnerable to the combined effects of a sedentary job and poor nutrition. The concept of exercise facilities at motorway service stations, vending machines selling fruit at depots and special truckers menus of soup and salad are a long way off, but it is these types of initiatives that are needed. When health promotion initiatives have been taken out to these groups of workers, they have been taken up – so it is not lack of interest which represents a barrier, but more lack of opportunity to make healthy choices.

KEY POINTS

- ∞ Promoting health needs programme planning and the assistance of many individuals within the business.
- ∞ A clear idea of the budget is essential before starting.
- ∞ Evaluation of the effectiveness is essential to secure further funding.
- ∞ Success is not easy to measure but it is likely that both qualitative (e.g. perceptions of likely changes to behaviour) and quantitative (e.g. numbers of people using the programme) measures will be needed.

Health promotion: the individual approach

'Be good to yourself. If you don't take care of
your body, where will you live?'

Kobi Yamada

The previous chapter dealt with health promotion in terms of changing the working environment and general interventions directed at individuals in groups rather than as individuals.

This chapter suggests ways in which, should resources allow, individuals can be helped to manage their weight.

The chapter will include possible ways of supporting people to maintain their weight as well as to effect weight loss and weight loss maintenance. From a public health perspective, huge benefits would accrue if people just failed to gain any more weight as they aged.

At an individual level, this means we need to concentrate on two types of person: the one who is not yet overweight but may become so and the one who is already overweight and obese.

FOR PEOPLE NOT YET OVERWEIGHT/OBESE

Biologically we put on weight as the decades pass, but for most people it is in the 40s and 50s that the weight gain becomes more noticeable and they complain of difficulty in losing weight. Providing education on how to keep active and eat healthily and watch for those extra pounds creeping on is the baseline intervention, which can be achieved in the workplace with little resource.

Suggestions for action include:
- encouraging everyone to know their BMI through health-focused weigh-in sessions

- charity fund-raisers (e.g. pay £1 to know your BMI – proceeds to Diabetes Research) and
- messages and information on notice boards.

Encouraging groups of people to come forward has distinct advantages – people who don't know their weight and people who have concerns both come forward as the approach is not personal.

Unless resources are more generous, this may be all that can be achieved but it is not insignificant, as people have to work at staying at the same weight they were in their 20s. Eating the same foods is likely to lead to weight gain and even obesity.

Getting started – engagement

It is now well recognised that motivators for men and women with regards to weight are very different. Studies suggest that if the target audience to be engaged is men, then emphasis needs to be placed on the importance of weight loss in 'getting fit'. Men often respond very differently to women when faced with the challenge of excess weight. They may have no history of dieting and very little knowledge of nutrition but are often able to focus and exert considerable will power to reach their goals.

Alternatively many women will have been trying many different diets over decades, some of which will have been successful, at least in the short term, but few will have managed to keep weight off for several years. In many cases they are interested in weight loss for the benefits of appearance, of easier to purchase and better fitting clothes, and of improved self-esteem and attractiveness. They are also concerned with health issues relating to themselves and their families.

This knowledge of the differences between audiences allows for the development of weight loss programmes specific to workplaces with different gender balances, as research suggests that the two groups do not necessarily mix well on the issue of dieting. It may be necessary to hold separate sessions to encourage participation by both men and women. Differences in ethnicity and the acceptability of combined gender groups will also be an issue in some workplaces where group approaches or individual approaches with shared learning are proposed.

FOR PEOPLE NOW OVERWEIGHT/OBESE

Many organisations want to help the people who have problems now or will have them in the future, and their wish is to focus resources on this selected group and make them the target audience for interventions.

But it is not always so easy. Getting people who have a weight problem to come forward can be difficult, as not everyone wants to face the issue personally and others feel the workplace is not the right setting for doing so.

When schemes start, it is best that they encourage voluntary participation with the hope that, when some people have success, others will be spurred on to join in.

Details of a possible workplace-based programme which could be carried out over eight weeks is shown in Appendix 4 but ground work needs to be undertaken prior to implementation of any programme.

All those involved in the programme (e.g. nurse, technician, administrator, catering staff) need to be clear on the current philosophy of weight management. This is to ensure consistency with healthcare professionals whom they may also consult (e.g. their GP).

The current philosophy has two basic principles:

▌ the aim is to no longer strive to 'ideal weight' (i.e. the middle of the BMI chart) but to attain realistic weight loss of 5–10% and
▌ to maintain it.

This may sound easy but it is deceptively difficult as, although many people can lose weight, over a period of 12 months the weight is regained.

The philosophy is at odds with many people's wishes to lose considerable amounts of weight and, in the case of females, to drop several dress sizes. This can be a latter goal once the initial 5–10% weight loss has been achieved, since setting small, progressive and realistic targets and celebrating their achievement is one of the techniques of successful weight loss. In does, however, mean that a key area of weight loss programmes is *management of expectations*.

RECRUITMENT OF INDIVIDUALS

Having identified the resources available and ensuring that they are adequate to sustain an individualised programme, the next step is recruitment. For the population-based approach this can be by emails, notices in canteen and rest rooms and word of mouth through the management chain. It is necessary to ensure adequate equipment is available and, most importantly, that there is a quiet and confidential area to measure and weigh people. A large mirror is also needed if waist circumference is to be measured. Sequential measurements should ideally take place at the same time of day each week and with the person wearing roughly the same clothing.

INITIAL ASSESSMENT

It is useful, if time allows, to take a history covering diets tried, successes and failures, and to look for suggestions of eating disorders such as binge and comfort eating. Then identify motivations and establish both the benefits and disadvantages of changing and of remaining the same – this can easily be done in a box drawing, as shown below:

Benefits of change	Disadvantages of change
Benefits of staying the same	Disadvantages of staying the same

FIGURE 9.1 Motivations chart.

Hopefully this demonstrates to the person that the advantages of taking some action outweigh the disadvantages. If they aren't persuaded, then consideration needs to be given to suggesting that perhaps it is not the right time to start the programme.

At the initial assessment, some key messages about nutrition need to be delivered. These include:

- small changes produce long-term results
- sugar should be replaced with saccharin tablets
- full-fat milk should be replaced with semi-skimmed or skimmed milk
- chips should be replaced with jacket potatoes
- behaviours leading to unhealthy eating need to be identified and cues removed to that behaviour
- the idea of 'being on a diet' needs to be replaced by that of 'adopting a healthy lifestyle'.

Set goals towards the 5–10% weight loss, losing 1–1.5 lb per week, and encourage sign-up by giving a co-operation card to each participant to bring with them every week.

One of the difficulties is in 'selling' the benefits of such a small weight loss. There is a lot of research which shows the reduced health risks associated with such a loss and this is another key message: 'You only need to lose a relatively small amount of weight to improve your health' and 'Losing more has further health benefits'.

Headline figures to support this, in relation to an obese person, include:

- loss of 5 kg reduces risk of type 2 diabetes by 50% (Manson *et al.* 1995)
- loss of 9 kg reduces diabetes-related deaths by 30–40% (Williamson *et al.* 1995)

▪ loss of 5% weight reduces fasting blood glucose by 15% (Dattilo and Krita-Etherton 1992)

▪ loss of 10–20% weight can stabilise blood sugar and improve life expectancy (Jung 1997).

ONGOING ASSESSMENT

Once participants are weighed, measured and have the key messages, it is necessary to provide ongoing support and assessment.

Some programme organisers ask participants to complete a *food diary* which demonstrates exactly how much is eaten in any one day over four to six weeks. This is useful if a person can not see how they can put on weight given what they believe they eat, and for the identification of cues and stressors which affect eating patterns.

It is important to be frank about the challenge of weight loss and weight maintenance – it is not easy and participants can become discouraged when the plateau of loss occurs at around three to four months. However, if they continue, further loss will occur as long as they review their calorie intake and make appropriate adjustments to their nutrition.

It is also important to warn participants about the temptations of *food marketing*, which aims to increase their consumption of calories, usually in the form of fats. Sometimes this is just misleading, as in cases where blatantly incorrect claims are made. However, the most familiar techniques of food marketing are 'super sizing' and 'meal deals', where buying more than the usual size of food or more than a food on its own is encouraged through the perception of a financial 'bargain'. Other techniques include 'buy one get one free' and snacks strategically positioned at supermarket checkouts. Participants need to be aware of all of these ways in which additional consumption of calories is promoted and resist them.

An example of the impact of a 'meal deal' over a sandwich and a 'super-sized' over a normal-sized burger meal is shown below.

Meal deal compared with sandwich alone
▪ **Sandwich alone** 400–500 calories
  Total calories: 400–500

Meal deal (sandwich plus soft drink plus crisps)
▪ sandwich 400–500 calories
▪ soft drink, e.g. branded Cola (can) 139 calories, 36.3 g sugar
▪ branded crisps 183 calories and 12.3 g fat
  Total calories: 722–822

In terms of the physical activity it would take to burn off just the *additional* calories (322–422), a person would have to walk an extra 8000 steps approximately to work off the sugary drink and crisps.

> **Super-sized compared with normal-sized burger meal**
> ▮ **Standard branded burger meal** consisting of
> ▮ large burger, regular 'fries' and regular branded soft drink
> ▮ 807 calories (includes 31.9 g fat and 38.3 g sugar)
>   Total calories: 807

> **Super-sized meal** consisting of
> ▮ large burger, super 'fries', super branded soft drink
> ▮ 1302 calories (includes 44.1 g fat and 91.3 g sugar)
>   Total calories: 1302

In terms of the physical activity it would take to burn off just the *additional* calories (495), a person would have to walk an extra 12 375 steps to work off the larger portions of burger, fries and soft drink.

MOTIVATING CHANGE

It is a controversial issue, but it may be better to spend time and effort with people who are most likely to succeed rather than with those with a 30-year history of dieting who 'eat nothing all day'.

What to do when there is 'no progress'

In the course of follow-up, it is necessary to provide support in terms of regular monitoring of progress and to make efforts to find positives and successes but not to support failure. For example, you might observe that while the participant has lost only one pound this week, their waist circumference has reduced two inches since they started. If someone fails to lose weight over a period of weeks or months there comes a time where the question has to be asked about the value of their continuation on the programme. Many dieters will wish to continue even though they have not made any changes to their lifestyle – it is enough for them that they are participating and being seen to be trying. This can be a difficult situation, but if it is made clear at the start of the programme that progress will be reviewed for everyone after three to four weeks and continuation will be based on results, then it is a fair way of allocating resources where they can be of most benefit with people who are actively taking steps to improve their health. Explaining to the person that they are perhaps 'not yet ready for this degree of change at this time' is one way of placing responsibility back on them and ensuring they are clear about the goals of the programme.

ASSESSING MOTIVATION

Assessing motivation and likelihood of success is also not easy but a structure which describes where people are on the path to behaviour change has been described by Prochaska and Diclemente.[1,2] They place people in one of several stages of readiness to change:

- pre-contemplation (the person does not admit to the need to change behaviour)
- contemplation (considering the possibility of change)
- preparation (making a decision to change but as yet not taking any action)
- action (changing the behaviour) and
- maintenance (adhering to the positive behaviour).

In theory, it should be easier to support a person in the preparation phase to lose weight than a person in the contemplation phase, but these stages are not linear and people move between them in short time spells.

What is clear from the psychological research is that, to be successful, weight loss programmes need to be individualised. Just giving information and advice is not enough. Lecturing people leads to the adoption of obstructive rather than change behaviours and should be avoided.

MOTIVATING DURING CONSULTATIONS

For occupational health practitioners, there may be opportunities to motivate people to adopt a healthy lifestyle during the course of consultations – e.g. statutory health surveillance or sickness absence reviews – rather than in a formal weight loss programme. In order to engage with workers, the following approach has been suggested:

- ask about their views on their weight
- advise on the link to potential health problems
- avoid confrontation through careful language (avoid 'You should . . .')
- dispel urban myths (e.g. that a person needs to lose weight down to a 'normal' BMI in order to get any benefit).

If a person has hypertension and is obese, the tailored message may include the fact that a 10 kg weight loss can reduce systolic blood pressure by 10 mg and diastolic by 20 mmHg (SIGN Guidelines). For a type 2 diabetic, the message may signal that the same loss could lead to a halving of fasting blood glucose (SIGN) or a 1 kg weight loss. In either case it could be mentioned that the loss would increase life expectancy by 3–4 months.

SUMMARY

The aims of health promotion at the individual level are:
- to help those who are not overweight to remain so
- to help those who are overweight not to become obese
- to help those who are overweight and obese to lose some weight
- to help maintain weight loss through an understanding of the mechanisms of weight gain, how this is slow and often imperceptible and how it can be managed.

When dealing with individuals, there are several key overall messages which need to be communicated, both in verbal and written forms.
- Weight loss is a complex issue.
- Weight gain is a result of genes and the environment.
- We cannot change our genes but we can change our environment.
- People do not become overweight and obese overnight; it's the steady almost daily excess of calories taken in over calories burnt off which leads to weight gain.
- Weight loss should not occur quickly, as the evidence suggests that steady weight loss is more likely to be sustainable than rapid loss, e.g. half a stone or more in a week is likely to be rapidly regained.
- If someone is obese then the loss of just 5–10% of body weight brings about huge reductions in risk factors for heart attacks and strokes.
- Diets don't work because people don't stick to them.
- Crash diets don't work because people lose water not fat. Crash dieting increases the risk of developing gallstones and osteoporosis and should be avoided.
- Managing weight is about making permanent lifestyle changes not dieting.
- Small changes to daily routines bring about big benefits in terms of weight loss.
- The aim should be to lose 1–1.5 lb per week and to keep that weight off.
- Good nutrition does more than just aid weight loss. Increasing the fruit and vegetables in the diet reduces the risk of strokes and heart disease and the correct mineral balance helps to prevent osteoporosis.
- Increasing your level of physical activity not only helps keep weight off but, in the longer term, it also reduces hypertension, cholesterol and osteoporosis.

CASE STUDY 9.2

The Work Fit initiative was devised by the Men's Health Forum for British Telecom (BT) and was launched for UK-based BT staff in September 2005. Following an internal media campaign that began in June, prospective participants were invited to register for Work Fit from early September and the first weekly task was sent out on 26 September. In all, 16 tasks were to be sent out, the last in mid-January 2006. Taken together, the 16 tasks amounted to a significant but achievable lifestyle improvement programme. Broadly, participants who followed the programme would significantly increase their physical activity levels, improve their diet and lose weight if appropriate.

By mid-November 2005, over 16 000 men and women had registered for Work Fit (about 18% of the UK-based workforce), a much higher number than originally anticipated. The proportion of male participants varied from about 60–75% depending on the age group, but middle-aged overweight men appear to have been particularly responsive. This level of male involvement is a significant achievement given men's general reluctance to engage with health issues, not least related to weight. The data also suggested that participation broadly reflects the demographic make-up and geographical distribution of BT's various lines of business.

As well as receiving weekly tasks by email, linked to supporting information on the BT intranet, participants could request personal support from a 'lifestyle adviser' (a nurse) by email. About 500 people used this service. About 10 000 people also received a free pedometer and 2500 of these were additionally sent a tape measure (to check waist circumference), a specially designed health information booklet and other written health information.

Participants registered with Work Fit as individuals or as a member of a team. Over 500 teams registered. They competed against each other to see which was achieving the greatest lifestyle change. This competition element was developed to encourage sustained participation, especially among men.

Each week, participants were asked to return two key pieces of data: their waist circumference and their total number of steps, as measured by a pedometer. The data already available at the time of writing suggested that many people had already lost significant amounts of weight, however researchers felt it was clearly too early to draw firm conclusions about the effectiveness of the programme. Work Fit ended in January 2006 and was followed by a three-month follow-up of participants to see whether the programme has resulted in sustained lifestyle improvement.

At the time of writing, data based on the 2170 participants (75% male) who it is known participated in Work Fit for two months or more showed that the mean weight loss was 1.9 kg and mean waist circumference for this group fell by 1.8 cm. The proportion of the group who fell into the normal weight category increased by almost 6%, while the proportion which was overweight fell by 4% and the proportion which was obese fell by almost 1%.

A full report on the Work Fit programme is available on the Men's Health Forum website from late in 2007 (www.menshealthforum.org.uk). Case study reproduced with kind permission of the Men's Health Forum.

KEY POINTS

∞   Small changes bring big results.

∞   Concentrate on improving both diet and nutrition.

∞   Be aware of techniques of food marketing.

∞   Losing weight steadily keeps it off – crash diets usually lead to rapid weight gain.

∞   Increasing physical activity also has benefits for cardiovascular and bone health.

REFERENCES

1 Prochaska JO, Di Clemente CC. Stages and processes of self change of smoking: toward an integrative model of change. *J Consult Clin Psychol.* 1983; **51**(3): 390–5.

2 Prochaska JO, Di Clemente CC, Norcross JC. In search of how people change: applications to addictive behaviours. *Am Psychol.* 1992; **47**: 1102–14.

CHAPTER 10

Legal aspects of obesity and the *Disability Discrimination Act*

'Discriminating against somebody because of his or her height, weight, hairstyle or something of that nature may not be a reasonable basis for making an employment decision, but that doesn't mean it's an unlawful basis.'

AC GOLDBERG, LAWYER, US[4]

Obesity has been defined as a medical condition for over 40 years. It is listed under the World Health Organizations International Classification of Diseases (ICD) as E.66. This recognition of obesity as a disease and a medical condition has implications for the way in which obese people are treated in the workplace.

Attention needs to be given to the consequences of obesity in causing disability. The *Disability Discrimination Act 1995* (DDA) requires that employers make reasonable adjustments to allow disabled people to obtain and remain in work. There are several key definitions within the Act. Disability is defined as a 'physical or mental impairment, which has a substantial effect on a person's day to day activities'. Day-to-day activities includes self-care and mobility.

The Act applies at all stages of employment: recruitment, promotion, opportunities for training and selection for redundancy. It requires that all employers (prior to 2005 it only applied to those with more than 15 employees) consider a disabled person and ensure that they are not directly or indirectly discriminated against.

SO ARE OBESE PEOPLE DISABLED?

The answer is not invariably but sometimes. There are two main situations where obesity may lead to disability, either directly (as a consequence of weight) or indirectly (as a consequence of co-morbidities).

Direct

There is no direct correlation between body mass index and disability or between body mass index and impaired mobility. The impact of excess weight on mobility occurs due to several variables including age, co-existing osteoarthritis and respiratory capacity. The longer a person has been obese, the more likely the obesity will have created abnormal forces on their knees, making osteoarthritis more likely. Obesity itself also carries with it an increased risk of osteoarthritis through a general effect over and above that of mechanical forces directly on knee joints. This is why obese people have an increased risk of osteoarthritis in non-weight-bearing joints such as the thumb. Finally, the deposition of fat in the thorax and the pressure on the lungs can impair respiratory capacity and lead to reduced exercise tolerance and impaired mobility.

Indirect

Obesity may indirectly cause problems with mobility through reduced cardiac output, strokes and the complications of diabetes. In these cases, obesity will be the underlying condition but it will be the complications which are sited as the cause.

REASONABLE ADJUSTMENTS

The DDA requires employers to make reasonable adjustments to allow disabled people to be in employment. But what are reasonable adjustments for an obese person?

A key point is the definition of what constitutes 'reasonableness'. Employers are not required to go to extreme lengths to adjust their workplaces or the work tasks but they must make 'reasonable' changes. Only the employment tribunals can decide what is reasonable; this is not the job of doctors, patients or their representatives and no cases have, to date, been before tribunals, but some suggestions are outlined below.

Adjustments to the workplace

Employers may need to consider changes to:
- arrange for business-class, rather than economy-class, travel (to ensure greater seat size and leg room)
- provide larger chairs for office work
- provide adjustable height desks to allow for clearance of larger thighs
- provide chairs with enhanced weight-bearing capacity.

Employers will need to pay particular attention to evacuation procedures, as evacuation chairs may not be appropriate because of size of the person and consequently if staff are expected to move an obese colleague down stairs there may be an attendant risk of musculoskeletal injury. In these circumstances, a safe haven approach maybe needed. Consultation with the local fire safety officer is needed to identify the safest approach and to take into account one or more staff with excess weight that may need specific policies and procedures.

Adjustments to the work tasks

Changes to work tasks can, inadvertently, exacerbate the problem of obesity. It may be tempting, when faced with an employee with mobility problems, to provide them with a parking space near the entrance, to exclude them from participating in activities which require physical activity and to make their working lives less active. But this is directly contrary to the medical advice they are receiving. Medically, the cornerstone of obesity management is to increase physical activity and reduce calorie intake. This conflict needs sensitive handling and discussion with the employee. Far more useful than reducing opportunities for physical activity is to work with the employee to support them in their efforts to reduce their weight. How this is done will depend on the individual and the employer.

CASE STUDY 10.1

PG is a 44-year-old man with a BMI of 45 kg/m^2. He had a physically active job which involved walking around six miles per day. He had a two-week holiday and then returned to work. His line manager noted that he appeared to be having difficulty walking around and was easily out of breath. This meant that he was much slower than usual in completing the tasks. He discussed the issue with Mr G and relocated him to a back office where he dealt with paperwork and general office tasks. Over the next four months Mr G's weight increased by 4 stone and he found himself in danger of losing his job as he had lost flexibility regarding jobs within the business.

The job relocation was undertaken in good faith but aggravated the problem. A similar outcome would have been found if he had been provided, in a well-intentioned way, with a motorised golf buggy to do his rounds. A more positive approach would have been to arrange a graded return-to-work programme involving increasing the distance walked on a daily basis, regular reviews and keeping up an active lifestyle during future vacations.

CASE STUDY 10.2

KW is a 38-year-old secretary with a BMI of 50 kg/m^2. She is able to access the office in which she works only via an elevator to the third floor but is unable to climb up or down stairs due to breathlessness caused by obesity. Her physical size also means that it would be difficult for anyone to pass her on the stairs. She is too heavy for the evacuation chair and her weight means that there is a high risk of back strain should she need to be evacuated when the lifts are out of use. With consultation with the local fire officer, a procedure is established whereby she moves to a safe haven on one of the landings for both fire drills and in event of a real fire.

But it is not just anti-disability discrimination law which may be breached with wrongful treatment of obese employees: in the UK, the Post Office recently lost an unfair dismissal claim brought by a 25-stone postman. He had been dismissed on health grounds after his weight suddenly increased. He was removed from delivery duties and his employer could not find a suitable alternative position. He was awarded £24 000 compensation and was reinstated as a postman when medical reports found him fit to work. The tribunal found that, given the size and resources of the organisation, the attempts to find an alternative role to accommodate his medical condition were inadequate and his dismissal through retirement on the grounds of ill-health was unreasonable and unfair.[1] Legal opinion is that employers cannot just sack or dismiss employees because they are obese, rather the employers would have to show the impact of the person's size on the business.[2] In the US, some courts have ruled that the morbidly obese – people who weigh more than twice as much or 100 pounds more than their optimal weight – are protected under disability law. But even if they are not disabled, disability law may protect them if their employer perceives them to be impaired. There is a strong overlap with other types of discrimination and bias. Thus an employer who fails to employ a woman for a job because she is overweight may be accused of gender discrimination if they recruit overweight men to the same role. Any job-related weight or fitness requirements need to carefully take account of both gender and ethnic differences or else specific groups may be disadvantaged and claim discrimination.[3]

Michigan, in the US, has led the way in discrimination legislation – not just on obesity but also on height and national origin. It has a specific statutory prohibition against employment discrimination based on weight. The Michigan statute reads: 'An employer shall not . . . fail or refuse to hire or recruit, discharge or otherwise discriminate against an individual with respect to employment, compensation, or a term, condition or privilege of employment, because of religion, race, colour, national origin, height, weight or marital status.'[4] One US legal opinion summarised the likely changes to legal protection against obesity discrimination: 'The language of state anti-discrimination statutes may be broadened to specifically include weight as one of the categories deserving legislative as well as judicial protection.'[5]

There is no doubt that, as the population increases in size, legal cases are establishing the basis of how employers are expected to behave, almost on a monthly basis. In the UK, not all cases get to court and public access to judgments. But we benefit from hearing about cases being treated internally under company procedures.

One such case is that of a 30-stone man who was dismissed from his job for being overweight and who is taking his case to the final stages of an internal company appeal. His employer maintained that he was too fat to undertake his role as he could not fit through security turnstiles or into his decontamination suit.[6] He argues he is being unfairly treated – we await the outcome with interest.

To date there have not been any cases which discuss the issue of whether an employer can require an overweight or obese person to lose weight. Would it even be ethical and acceptable to write into an employment contract the need to remain a certain size or not exceed a certain weight? Already some employers are looking at requiring employees to watch their weight. It has been reported that Air India has told cabin crew to lose weight or risk being grounded (presumably with loss of pay due to flights not worked). They justify the action saying that they want to improve the image of staff by encouraging fitness and better eating. No mention is made of what an ideal weight is or whether any crew have yet been grounded.[7]

KEY POINTS

- ∞   Obesity is a recognised medical condition.
- ∞   Obese people may have mobility problems and difficulty with lifting.
- ∞   Prejudice and discrimination still exists for this group.
- ∞   The courts have yet to test the concept that obese people are covered by the DDA, but the condition meets (in the opinion of the author) the criteria.

REFERENCES

1 Sheppherd and Wedderburn. Reported in *Employment Law Update*. 1 February 2005 (www.capita-ld.co.uk accessed 2 February 2005).

2 Chamberlain J, Fielding J. Care needed when tackling obesity in the workplace. Employment Law. *Birmingham Post*. 20 May 2005.

3 Goldberg AC. Workplace obesity raises complex legal questions (Discrimination). *HR Briefing*. 1 July 2002; **3**(1).

4 *Mich. Comp. Laws*. Ann sec. 37.2102.

5 Johnson T. Analysis of weight based discrimination: obesity as a disability. *Labor Law Journal*. 1995; **46**(4): 238–44.

6 *The Times*. 1 February 2005, reported in *Employment Law Update*. 1 February 2005 (www.capita-ld.co.uk accessed 2 February 2005).

7 Delhi bellies. *The Times*. 15 April 2005.

CHAPTER 11

Further resources

> 'Every human being is the author of
> their own disease.'
>
> S SIVANANDA (1887–1963)

BOOKS

Ewles L, Simnett I. *Promoting Health: a practical guide*. 3rd ed. Middlesex, England: Scutari Press; 1995.

Fletcher GL, Grundy SM, Hayman L, editors. *Obesity: impact on cardiovascular disease*. Oxford: Blackwell Publishing; 1999.

Kopelman PG and Stock M, editors. *Clinical Obesity*. Oxford: Blackwell Publishing; 1998.

O'Donnell MP. *Health Promotion in the Workplace*. 3rd ed. New York: Delmar; 2001. A framework for studying health promotion which reviews the findings of the last decade.

Wilkinson C. *Fundamentals of Health at Work: the social dimensions*. London: Taylor & Francis; 2001. Describes an integrated approach to workplace health including health and safety, occupational health and health promotion.

FURTHER READING

Nature Insight 2000; **404**. Dedicated issue outlining medical aspects of obesity, including genetics and treatment.

ARTICLES AND DOCUMENTS

Making women and girls more active – a good practice guide. Sport Scotland. Published 7 December 2005. Available from Sport Scotland in hard copy or as a pdf to download from www.sportscotland.gov.uk

At least five a week – evidence of the impact of physical activity and its relationship to health. A report from the Chief Medical Officer. Department of Health. London: Department of Health; 2004.

The management of obesity and overweight. An analysis of reviews of diet, physical activity and behavioural approaches. Evidence briefing. Health Development Agency. London: Department of Health; 2003. Also available at www.had.nhs.uk/evidence

Pumping up the pressure: a qualitative evaluation of a workplace health promotion initiative for male employees. Lomas and McCluskey. *Health Educ J.* 2005; **64**: 88–95.

Exercise and the bottom line: promoting physical and fiscal fitness in the workplace. A commentary. NA DiNubile, C Sherman. *The Physician and Sports Medicine* February 1999; **27** (2).

WEBSITES – GOVERNMENTAL

General

www.doh.gov.uk/stats/trends Government trend data.

www.nao.gov.uk/publications/reports UK National Audit Office report into costs of obesity to the NHS and cross-governmental initiatives (report 1220).

www.healthpromotionagency.org.uk Health Promotion Agency, Northern Ireland.

www.nice.org UK National Institute of Clinical Excellence (NICE) guidance on use of drugs and surgery in obesity.

www.cdc.gov US Centers for Disease Control, Atlanta.

www.nhlbi.nih.gov/guidelines/obesity/ob-gdlns.pdf Evidence-based report on all aspects of obesity.

www.signupweb.net Government initiatives on healthy workplaces.

www.had-online.org.uk/downloads/pdf/obesity-evidence-briefing.pdf Evidence-based reviews of obesity management.

www.health-challenge@wales.gsi.gov.uk An excellent site with a range of supporting resources and guidance for media, schools, workplaces etc.

Nutritional information

www.food.gov.uk UK Government's Food Standards Agency. Information on food safety and a section on diet and health includes discussion of 'food myths'. Also provides advice on diet and nutrition.

www.eatwell.gov.uk Eatwell website, including information on healthy catering and a sample customer satisfaction questionnaire to assess views of employees.

ww.health-challenge@wales.gsi.gov.uk Good practice guide on healthy eating for meetings and events.

Physical activity

www.sportengland.org UK Government body provides advice on being active and includes a search facility for local sports centres and facilities in England. Operates via regional offices.

www.sportscotland.org.uk Responsible for developing sport and physical activity in Scotland.

www.sports-council-wales.co.uk Responsible for encouraging physical activity in the natural environment. Provides information on Metro Allan, a UK lottery-funded project on increasing activity in the south Wales valleys through increased walking.

www.healthchallengewales.gov.uk Country-wide campaign to promote health in Wales, including through increased physical activity. Free action pack available on Tel. 0845 606 4050.

WEBSITES – NON-GOVERNMENTAL

General

www.bbc.co.uk/bigfatproblem

www.bhf.org British Heart Foundation. Includes statistics, graphs and material for presentations.

Evidence-based research

www.jr2.ox.ac.uk/bandolier Research and systematic reviews of obesity management.

www.nelh.nhs.uk National Electronic Library for Health.

www.phel.gov.uk Public Health Electronic Library. One-stop shop for public health information. Has search function for organisations, events and web resources.

www.nationalobesityforum.org Primary care interest group, includes primary care management protocol for obesity.

Nutritional information

www.bda.uk.com British Dietetic Association. Website for UK-registered dieticians. Includes the 'Desktop Dietician' which provides free advice on diet, nutrition and lifestyle. Also provides information on the latest food facts on popular diets such as the GI diet.

www.nutrition.org.uk Outlines nutritional aspects of various foods. Includes a PowerPoint presentation on healthy eating which can be downloaded. Contains section on nutrition and health, covering such topics as diet and cancer, vegan and vegetarian diets. Also provides guidance on food labelling.

www.thinkvegetables.co.uk Provides information on which vegetables are in season and recipes.

www.weightloss.co.uk Provides an outline of various diets from Atkins to the Grapefruit diet.

Physical activity help and support

www.urbanwalks.co.uk Commercial consultancy service providing leaflets outlining home and office exercises, posters to encourage use of stairs and information for display in lifts.

www.sustrans.org.uk Organisation which aims to increase walking in daily life. Provides free cycle maps and produces a 'cycle-friendly employers' factsheet.

www.sports-council-wales.co.uk Information on national initiatives and on particular sports.

Professional associations

www.hpw.org Health Professions Wales. In English and Welsh, offering careers information and HPW publications and events.

www.bhf.org British Heart Foundation. Varied web resource including graphs and data on heart disease in the UK. Think Fit action pack contains workplace activity planners, facts and figures, ideas and challenges. Also includes an activity wall planner and a Think Fit tee-shirt. Details of cost from Tel. 0870 600 6566 or www.bhf/thinkfit

PRACTICAL HELP FOR EMPLOYEES

www.bbc.co.uk/bigchallenge BBC website containing information and advice on diet and exercise. Includes a free online health club and with a free assessment and a six-week diet and exercise plan.

www.pathstohealth.org.uk supports local schemes in Wales to promote walking in the community. Group-led walks and information about safe, accessible places locally. Tel. 01259 218 855.

www.whi.org.uk Walking the Way to Health. Joint initiative from British Heart Foundation, The Countryside Agency and Countryside Council for Wales, to encourage use of countryside by communities. Organises guided walks, sets up signposted paths and trains volunteers as walk leaders. Website provides details of local walks.

Patient groups and guidance

www.wlsinfo.org.uk Weight-loss surgery patient support and information line. Tel. 0151 222 4737.

www.dlf.org.uk The Disabled Living Foundation has produced a factsheet on choosing equipment for heavier people weighing 30 stone plus. It can be downloaded free of charge from the website at www.dlf.org.uk/factsheets and provides guidance on where to go for help to buy chairs, beds, mobility aids and footwear, and on diet and exercise. Tel. 020 7289 6111 extn 211. Helpline: 0845 130 9177.

Common questions and answers

Q. Would liposuction reduce my abdominal fat and risk of heart disease/ diabetes etc.?

A. No. Liposuction removes only subcutaneous fat so abdominal liposuction would not affect the stores of dangerous fat in the abdomen itself. The only way to get rid of this fat is to eat fewer calories and exercise more.

Q. Can reducing salt help me lose weight?

A. In theory, yes. When salt is taken into the body, water passes with it so the body carries excess water which can cause not only weight gain but also raised blood pressure and risk of stroke and heart attacks.

Q. How can I make simple changes to reduce salt in my diet?

A. You could try changes such as:
- removing salt from the table
- adding salt to food only after tasting
- considering low-salt substitutes
- trying to substitute commoner foods for low-salt alternatives:
  - bread replaced by Matzos
  - fruit and fibre replaced by puffed wheat
  - cornflakes replaced by sugar-free natural muesli
  - dry-roasted peanuts replaced by fruit
  - tinned tomato soup replaced by tomato and basil salad
  - crisps replaced by dried fruit or dry non-salted nuts.

Q. How much should I lose and how quickly?

A. Aim to lose 1–1.5 lb per week. Loss at this rate is less likely to be regained and more likely to stay off.

Q. I have seen a diet in a woman's magazine that claims you can lose one stone in one week. Will it work for me?

A. Most 'lose a stone in a week' diets don't work, as, if you reduce your calorie intake drastically, you lose water not fat and rapidly regain any weight lost. It is better to lose weight slowly and keep it off.

Q. Do diets work?

A. In the short term, most diets will lead to weight loss but the problem is that many are restrictive and people don't find it easy to stick to them and quickly return to eat their usual food. It is better to not go on a diet but to make permanently healthy lifestyle changes. If you are not on a diet you cannot come off it and lapse!

Food labelling

ENERGY

Energy is measured in calories (kcal) and is shown on foods as kcal per 100 g of the product.

Healthy daily amount: for women, 2000 calories; for men, 2500 calories.

FAT

Total fat is given per 100 g of product.

Examples: 20 g of fat per 100 g is a lot of fat; 3 g of fat per 100 g is a small amount of fat.

Healthy daily amount: maximum 70 g per day for women; 90 g for men.

Saturated fat

Examples: 3 g of saturated fat per 100 g is a lot; 1 g of saturated fat per 100 g is a small amount.

Healthy daily amount: no more than 20 g per day for women; 30 g for men.

SUGAR

Not always included on labels but the higher the term 'sugar' appears on the list of contents, then the more in the product.

Examples: 10 g of sugar per 100 g is a lot; 2 g of sugar per 100 g is a small amount.

Healthy daily amount: no more than 7 teaspoons per day for women; 8 teaspoons per day for men.

PROTEIN

Examples: there are no official figures as to what constitutes a lot and what constitutes a small amount of protein.

Healthy daily amount: 45 g of protein per day for women; 56 g of protein per day for men.

SODIUM

By law, amounts of salt must be on labels but it is sometimes called 'salt' and sometimes 'sodium chloride'.

Healthy daily amount: no more than 2.5 g per day for men or women. (Note: Convert sodium to salt by multiplying by 2.5.)

THINGS TO BE AWARE OF

- Manufacturers have a leeway of plus or minus 20% in their description of calories.
- 'Low-fat spreads' mean they contain 3 g per 100 g or less. There is no such thing as a genuinely low-fat spread.
- 'Lite' refers to the texture of a product not its calorie count.
- 'Fat-free' does not mean low-calorie or calorie-free – watch the sugar and carbohydrate content.
- Some 'lower-fat' products refer to the difference in fat content between regular and low-fat alternatives of the same product – this does not mean that they are 'low-fat'.

For further information: *What Are You Really Eating? How to become label-savvy*. Amanda Ursell. (Hay House £5.99)

Popular diets, past and present

'There is no love sincerer than the love of food.'

Newcastle Airport restaurant, 19 May 2006

1960s
Banana diet
Very strict, low-calorie diet of bananas and a lot of salad. The banana provided a source of slow-release carbohydrate and was supposed to fill you up and stop sugar cravings.

1967
Weight Watchers diet
Weight Watchers arrived in the UK from the US and provided a system of regulating intake through setting a limit on the number of points of food which could be eaten in a day. Successful, healthy, it remains today as one of the major commercial slimming organisations.

1968
Bread and butter diet
Yes, only bread and butter were allowed to be eaten, but in a calorie-controlled way.

1969
Ayds tablets
Chewy, carbohydrate lumps resembling fudge were to fill up the stomach, however, some people found that the taste made them crave food.

1973
Beverley Hills diet
One of the first trendy diets to sweep through whole countries and also one of the first to require a book purchase to describe the philosophy and how to follow it. The diet advocated eating pineapple before every meal to break down fat. Still followed today by some enthusiasts but no evidence it works.

1979 (although it originally also appeared in the 1950s)
Grapefruit diet
Grapefruit were thought to curb the appetite. It was believed that grapefruit, as slow releasers of carbohydrate, would, when regularly consumed throughout the day, lead to flatter levels of sugars in the body. There is no evidence it works.

1983
F-plan diet
High-fibre diet focusing on making you feel full so you ate less and restricted calorie intake. It has stood the test of time and an updated version has recently been released.

1984
Rosemary Conley's hip and thigh diet
Nutritionally balanced, low-fat menus combined with exercise produced slow, steady weight loss. Remains popular today.

1985
Slimfast
This involved replacing two meals per day with protein shakes or cereal bars. Has been proven to work in tests and has its own set of followers who like shakes and the simplicity of the programme.

1989
Cambridge diet
A meal replacement diet from the US which includes high-protein, low-fat soups, meal bars and milk shakes. To follow the diet it is necessary to join a club and so communal support has been a feature of this successful scheme.

1991
Cabbage soup diet
Initially described in the 1980s, it took a decade to reach UK shores. Based on eating as much cabbage soup as you liked, with other high-fibre and low-fat foods, it was essentially a very low-calorie diet. Produced rapid, short-term weight loss but, like many such diets, was very difficult to sustain and so had a high drop-out rate.

1997
Atkins diet

A low-carbohydrate eating plan which had been around for years but had a second surge of interest in the late 1990s. Heavily criticised by the medical and dietary establishment, it was a favourite particularly with men who enjoyed fried breakfasts and still lost weight. Many followers found that what was initially very exciting – to eat foods previously thought of as 'naughty and forbidden' – actually became monotonous and boring. Few people sustained the diet for long, although the results for the first few months were often impressive. The jury is out on how Atkins leads to weight loss, as the food consumed tends to be high-fat and high-calorie. Theories include the high protein content promoting satiation and so smaller appetites and the ketotic state of the body somehow consuming more calories.

1999/ 2000
Zone diet

A diet plan involving balanced protein, carbohydrate and fat intake and focusing on foods which reportedly affect the hormonal balance. Never really one of the major diet fads in the UK, but some followers remain enthusiastic.

2003
South Beach diet

A sensible diet plan which is marketed as a lifestyle change rather than a diet. Followers eat the healthiest carbohydrates, fats and proteins. Not a struggle to follow and not disliked by the professional dietician community.

2005
GI diet

The GI (glycaemic index) diet works as a method of weight loss by keeping blood sugar levels stable, which in turn keeps hunger under control. The theory is that rapid surges of sugar into the bloodstream, such as come after drinking a can of sweetened soft drink, lead to output of insulin which stimulates the appetite. Low-GI foods release carbohydrate slowly and so, with stable blood sugar levels, there are no insulin and appetite surges.

Low-GI diets have been associated with a number of healthy benefits, but research has been limited. Most of it concentrates on diabetes and cardiovascular disease and there is some evidence that following a GI diet can benefit lipid levels[1] and lower insulin after meals.[2] There have been inconsistent results reported in cancer studies[3] and no evidence to suggest that a low-GI diet is better than a high-GI diet for long-term weight control.

There are limitations to the use of the diet.

■ The GI value of a food can be affected by processing and state of ripeness of fruit and vegetables.

■ GI information is limited to individual foods and there is a lack of information on the effects of combining foods.

■ The number of foods listed as either high or low is not always consistent with current healthy eating messages. Thus bananas are high GI, whilst some biscuits and cakes are low GI.

■ GI only focuses on the carbohydrate in a food and not on its other nutrients.

■ Lack of consistent, accurate food labelling can make making choices based on GI difficult.

REFERENCES

1 Frost G *et al*. Glycaemic index as a determinant of serum HDL-cholesterol concentration. *Lancet*. 1999; **353**: 1045–8.

2 Wolever TM, Jenkins DJ, Vuksan V, *et al*. Beneficial effect of a low glycaemic index diet in type 2 diabetes. *Diabet Med*. 1992; **9**: 451–8.

3 World Cancer Research Fund. Informed 18. GI – just another fad diet? Summer 2005.

Suggested eight-week programme for weight loss in a workplace

COURSE PREPARATION BY THE WORKPLACE IN-HOUSE TEAM

▌ Identify a trained, keen dietician/nurse to lead the group. Ensure their availability over eight weeks and familiarity with programmes of this type. Dieticians should be registered with the British Dietetic Association. Some nurses may have had specialised training provided through their primary care trust and may be running clinics which are evaluated in their doctor's surgery. *Enthusiasm and a history of personal dieting is not enough to run a course.*

▌ Local information on physical activity opportunities is essential to facilitate take-up. Having to find out yourself is a barrier which many staff won't overcome. Look to the primary care trust health promotion teams to supply information on local health walks schemes, cycle paths, evening cycling clubs, 'green gyms' (local working parties that sustain environmental development) and any reduced-rate schemes for local gyms.

▌ Contact local restaurants and ask them to supply menus for scrutiny. Explain what the initiative is about and encourage them to label healthier options if they are not already doing so, thus making it easier for everyone to make the healthier choice.

▌ Develop a 'welcome pack' which describes each session so that participants know what to expect. A sample is shown below.

WELCOME PACK

Welcome to the Brueton Weight Loss Programme. All the sessions below are run by a registered dietician/nurse with specialised training. We aim to show you how to live a healthier lifestyle to help you lose weight.

Key points

■ You will be weighed at each session.
■ There will be a handout for each session.
■ You will have the opportunity to ask questions in the group at each session and on a one-to-one basis with the dietician/nurse after each session.
■ Once started, we ask that you commit to attend all eight sessions and complete the course.

Main objectives of the course

■ To enable you to identify current eating habits and life issues which are preventing you from eating healthily.
■ To help you understand the benefits of healthy eating and of physical activity.
■ To provide you with the skills and knowledge to help you lose weight by better understanding of food labelling and types of exercise.

Session 1 – Where are we now?

Covers the links between what we eat and our health. Includes completion of a nutrition questionnaire, taking weight and waist measurement, body mass index (BMI) calculation, target-setting and objectives.

Session 2 – What is healthy eating?

Covers making individual plans for change and guidelines for healthy eating, recognising good and bad foods and what we need to aim for in terms of calories and fat intake. Considers good substitutes for favourite unhealthy foods. Also what the ideal diet is, use of food diaries and the importance of portion size.

Session 3 – What is healthy activity?

Covers why exercise is good for us and for weight loss. Considers how to create that energy deficit and the successful maintenance of weight loss. Also how to access physical activity services locally, through the doctor and through public and private facilities.

Session 4 – Emotions and eating

Covers motivation, barriers to change, overcoming barriers, managing relapses.

Session 5 – Eating out

Covers how to plan to eat out – how to cope with eating out in Italian, French, Indian and Chinese restaurants. Considers the best selections from an average menu and how they compare in terms of calories and fat with the 'usual' healthy diet.

Session 6 – Understanding food labels

This is a practical session at the local supermarket. Covers identifying high-fat and high-sugar foods, awareness of the meaning of 'low-fat' and other misleading labels and claims made for foods. Also, identifying true low-fat, low-calorie alternatives.

Session 7 – Diets and why they don't work

An overview of the main approach of some of the more popular diets over the last few years and why they don't work in the longer term.

Session 8 – Evaluation: how was it for you?

Final weigh-in, check on progress and discussion regarding the next steps and maintenance of that weight loss. Tips on managing temptation and relapse. Explanation of the plateau effect of weight loss after two to three months of success and the need to keep to healthy eating and physical activity to overcome it.

Suggested healthy substitutions for traditional workplace buffet lunches

Traditional	Healthier option
sandwiches on white bread	wholemeal pitta parcels containing Mediterranean vegetables
	rice cakes with tuna and peppers
	rice cakes with low-fat cream cheese and either tomato or cucumber
	rice cakes with salmon, lemon and parsley
goujons	chicken on skewers with green and red peppers and onion sections
	roast beef and small onions on skewers
samosas	vegetarian kebabs (onions, mushrooms and courgettes on a skewer)
	wild rice and vegetable salad
crisps	carrot and courgette batons and cauliflower with a low-fat dip
gateau	fresh fruit
	fruit kebabs
	fruit salad
	low-fat yoghurts
cream cakes	variations on fruit (as above)

Examples of nutritional interventions and increased physical activity

NUTRITIONAL INTERVENTIONS

Canteen/restaurant

- Provide healthy options for all meal times and snacks.
- Label all food for fat/salt and indicate healthiest options.
- Offer grilled rather than fried food.
- Remove truly unhealthy food such as burgers and chicken nuggets.
- Restrict foods such as chips to once per week.
- Increase the availability of fresh fruit, salads and vegetables.
- Increase the availability of low-fat desserts such as yoghurts.
- Use the eating area as a site for delivering information about healthy eating and advertising such events as local farmers markets.
- Provide cookery demonstrations on easy-to-prepare healthy food.
- Identify if there is a market for healthy takeaway meals to reduce the stress of working then having to cook at home.
- Consider ways in which healthy options could be subsidised either by the employer or the supplier.
- Ensure that the canteen is bright, clean and airy.
- Ensure an adequate length of lunch break.
- Ensure that meals for shift workers are equally nutritious.

Vending facilities

- Ensure that any drinks vending machine contains at least 30% fruit juice and water.
- Substitute snack bars with fruit and energy snacks.
- Place unhealthy foods at the top and bottom of the display.

- Consider penalising unhealthy snacks and subsidising healthy ones.
- Ensure that vending facilities used by staff at night are well stocked with healthy choices.
- Surround the machine with healthy food messages on notice boards.
- Monitor usage and selection of healthy options and advertise positive changes on notice boards and in newsletters.
- Provide information on actual fat and calorie content of unhealthy options near to the machine along with benefits of healthier options. For example:
  - calories in can of Coke = about 140
  - calories in can of Diet Coke = 1.5
  - calories in can of 7-Up = about 145
  - calories in can of Diet 7-Up = 3.3

Sandwich and snack vendors

- Encourage the sale of healthier options only.
- Ensure provision of fruit and energy bars and that they are the most visible items on sale.
- If no sandwich vendor currently visits the workplace and people visit fast food outlets locally, ask several vendors to consider visiting to provide an alternative food source.

General food availability

Reception

- Remove sweets, possibly replacing them with fruit if the budget allows.

Meetings

- Remove sweets, mints and cordials from tables. Replace with plain still and sparkling water only.
- Consign a single bottle of cordial to the side of the room where it is accessible on request.
- Provide apples and other fruit on tables or at the side in full visibility of delegates.

Conferences

- Remove pastries on arrival. Either do not replace or substitute with single-piece fruit kebabs.
- Meals should be light, fixed-portion (either by food being plated or served) rather than a 'help yourself' buffet, and contain at least two healthy options in the hot food section.
- Ask that cheese, if served, be cut into small cubes of about 1 cm in diameter. This reduces portion size and makes an attractive display.

Sandwich lunches

▮ Talk to in-house and contract caterers about supplying rice cakes and pitta parcels rather than bread.

▮ If bread is served, ensure that it is wholegrain and that fillings are low in fat and salt.

▮ Ask about the availability of individualised salad pots with low-fat dressings.

Communal kitchens

▮ Provide clean, bright eating areas with good facilities.

Celebrations

▮ Encourage fresh fruit as a means of celebrating birthdays etc rather than cakes but beware as this maybe a sensitive area for staff.

Nutritional information

▮ Provide information in a variety of formats (e.g. hard copy, on intranet, in messages on pay slips, posters and flyers) and in a variety of locations, including the canteen.

▮ Consider more innovative places to display messages, such as the back of doors in toilets (females) or above the cistern (males).

▮ Use conventional notice boards and electronic messaging systems, the latter particularly for staff who work or are based offsite.

INCREASING PHYSICAL ACTIVITY

Getting to work

▮ Review transport policies and encourage greater use of cycling and public transport. Set up a transport system between two company sites, if feasible.

▮ Reward staff for giving up car parking spaces (financial, extra holidays etc.)

▮ If premises are located on a waterway, explore feasibility of water taxis or advertise canal towpath cycle routes.

▮ Advertise the number of steps taken towards a personal daily goal to be gained by parking furthermost away from the company entrance.

Getting around and about at work

▮ Encourage the use of stairs by siting swipe entry card systems at bottom of stairs.

▮ Slow down escalators so people feel it's quicker to walk.

▮ Encourage exercise by placing posters in lifts.

▮ Decorate and light stair wells so they are more inviting and consider adding piped music.

▮ Have a 'Lift-free Day' campaign.

■ Have meetings standing up.
■ If in an open plan environment, consider setting up a walking track around the perimeter.
■ Set out walking trails around the site or into the local town. Record the number of steps approximately which would be undertaken to complete the trail.
■ If space permits, ask local instructors to consider running tai chi or other classes at the workplace. These could be self-funded or subsidised.

'Out of office' work

■ Use public transport as much as possible – use the tube, coach, plane or train rather than driving (people walk more when using public transport).
■ Stay only in hotels with 'in-room gym' facilities or swimming pool, gym etc.
■ As a company, sponsor a football or netball team to play in the local leagues, or a group of employees to take part in a Fit Run.
■ Sponsor the run yourself to encourage participation.
■ Support a company Weight Loss Club, providing rewards for single employees or groups of employees who lose the biggest percentage of body weight. The reward could be a donation to the charity of workers' choice or a day off for them to work for the charity of their choice. Rewards do not need to be financial and can be coupled with corporate social responsibility initiatives and contacts.
■ Negotiate discounts for gym and sports membership with national chains.
■ Provide information on local walks, cycle paths and free sports 'samplers' at local leisure centres.

American College of Occupational and Environmental Medicine 2004 Labor Day checklist on obesity

Every year the American College of Occupational and Environmental Medicine (ACOEM) publishes a checklist outlining action which can be taken by employers and employees to combat major health issues. In 2004 this checklist addressed obesity and it is reproduced here with the permission of the ACOEM (*see also* their website, www.acoem.org).

2004 ACOEM LABOR DAY CHECKLIST

Controlling Obesity in the Workplace

This year, the American College of Occupational and Environmental Medicine's (**ACOEM's**) **Labor Day Checklist** deals with controlling **obesity** in the workplace.

Millions of Americans are fighting the battle against **obesity** – a health issue that can result in adverse or even fatal health outcomes, staggering healthcare costs, and reduced workplace productivity. It is important to remember that **obesity** goes beyond individual lifestyle choices, but that everyone can work to control this problem on a daily basis both in the workplace – where employers have an opportunity to provide a supportive environment that enables healthy lifestyle choices – and in the home. The 2004 **Checklist** provides several steps employers and employees can take to fight **obesity**.

For All Employers and Employees
Educational
Employers and employees alike should learn the basic principles of attaining and maintaining healthier weight. Implement a workplace wellness program that

123

provides mechanisms to aid employees in adopting healthy lifestyles. Encourage the formation of an employee wellness team. Provide educational material on the health risks of being overweight. Provide materials on how to eat healthier. Post a listing of calories expended for common activities such as walking, swimming, bicycling, and running. Participate in workplace wellness activities and read the educational material provided by your employer.

If your employer offers employee wellness teams, join the team!

Carefully read the nutritional and caloric content information on food labels.

Work Environment and Physical Activity

Employers can make the work environment a setting for policy changes that will lead to more physically active employees. Investigate alternative work schedules to minimize fatigue which can contribute to unhealthy eating habits. Consider having at least one casual dress day a week. A recent study found that when employees dressed casually, they were more physically active. Encourage the use of stairways instead of elevators by placing signs near the elevator and stairs highlighting the health benefits of stair use. Ensure that stairways are accessible and are properly illuminated. Discourage employees from eating at their desks. Even a short walk to the cafeteria/lunch room can be helpful. Support physical activity breaks during the work day. Allow employees enough time for lunch so that they can walk or use the gym. If stressed, do deep breathing exercises and practice these techniques instead of reaching for food. Wear comfortable shoes for walking. Use the stairs instead of an elevator whenever possible throughout the day. If possible, walk or bike to work. If you must drive, park your car in a spot farthest from the entrance to benefit from walking the extra distance. During breaks, get up and walk around the office or exercise. There are a variety of exercises that you can do at your desk. Walk at lunch – form an office walking club.

Food Choices

Employers can help promote sensible eating habits.

- Offer appealing, healthy choices in cafeterias and/or vending machines.
- Provide nutritional information for cafeteria selections. Smaller employers should encourage healthier food and beverages in cafeterias or vending machines.
- Provide healthier snacks at meetings and other employee events. For example, serve fruit, popcorn, and low-fat yogurt. Provide bottled water in the vending areas or cafeteria. Request healthier food choices be served in the cafeteria and provided in vending machines.
- Make fruit and other low-calorie, nutrient-rich products your food of choice.
- Make healthier selections at fast food restaurants such as salads with low-

calorie dressings.

▮ Drink water instead of soft drinks or other high sugar beverages.

For large to mid-size employers

Consider offering memberships or discounts to health clubs. Offer wellness classes on nutrition, exercise, and weight management. Provide worksite walking paths and bike racks. Utilize health club memberships offered by employers. Enroll in exercise, nutrition, and/or weight management classes.

General guidance

▮ Before starting a diet and/or exercise program, consult with your physician. If you experience a sudden weight gain or loss, see your doctor immediately.

▮ Have a glass of water before meals to fill your stomach and reduce your desire for food.

▮ Avoid purchasing high-caloric or high-sugar food items. Have fruit, vegetables, and healthy snacks readily available in the home.

▮ Eat dinner as early as possible. Calories will have more time to burn off prior to bedtime.

▮ Limit your portion size when eating at home or in a restaurant, and never supersize your food order.

▮ Do not drive to places that are within easy walking distance. Walking helps to control weight.

▮ Get off the couch and start walking or become involved in a sport or other activity such as gardening. Make it your goal to engage in at least 30 minutes of moderate physical activity each day.

▮ Exercise with a friend – it's more fun and motivating!

©ACOEM 2004 Labor Day Checklist
www.acoem.org

Index

abdominal fat 8–10
accountants 81–2
ACOEM Labor day Checklist 123–5
activities of daily living (ADL) 20
aerobic capacity 25
age and obesity 24
agility issues 25
airlines 38, 97
Alzheimers disease 18
angina 19
anticonvulsants 13
antidepressants 13
antidiscrimination legislation 31, 32–3,
    93–7
antihistamines 13
antipsychotics 13
appetite regulation 12–13
    medical approaches 47–8
aprons and overclothes 26, 55
Asian populations, obesity definitions
    8–10
assessment of individuals 85–8
asthma 18
Atkins diet 111
attitudes towards obese people 31–5
attractiveness studies 31–2
Ayds tablets 109

banana diet 109
Beverley Hills diet 110
binge eating syndrome 19
BMI (body mass index) 7–10
    and diabetes risk 16

body fat estimations 10
bread and butter diet 109
breast cancer 18
British Dietetic Association weight loss
    programmes 113–15
British Telecom (BT), Work Fit initiative
    90–1
Brueton Weight Loss Programme
    113–15
business needs 2–6

cabbage soup diet 110
call centre work 28
    workplace interventions 78–80
Cambridge diet 110
cancers 18
cardiovascular disease 17
cardiovascular fitness 25
chairs and desks 26
Choosing Activity: a physical activity
    action plan (DoH 2005) 45
Choosing Health: making healthy choices
    easier (DoH 2004) 4
colon cancer 19
contraceptive drugs 13
Cook vs Rhode Island Department of
    Mental Health, Retardation and
    Hospitals ruling 32–3
coronary heart disease (CHD) 17
corporate social responsibility (CSR)
    55–6
corticosteroids 13
cosmetic surgery 50

costs for workplace interventions
   large budget options 64–6
   low budget options 61–4
   no budget options 58–61
CSR *see* corporate social responsibility
customer reactions 37
cycling 61–3

delivery workers 82
dementia 18
demographic changes 2–3
   prevalence of obesity 1
design of work activities 69–73
diabetes 15–17
diet composition
   general advice 42
   see also nutrition and diet education
diet types 109–12
Disability Discrimination Act-1995
   93–7
   case studies 95–6
   definitions 93–5
discrimination and prejudice issues 2,
   31–8
   attitudes and challenges 31–5
   impact on healthcare access 36–7
   personal accounts 38
   public and customer responses 37
dismissal from work 96–7
Dole Food Company Inc. (California)
   64–5
drug therapies 46–8
   Orlistat 47
   Rimonabant 48
   Sibutramine 47
drugs causing obesity 13

economic costs
   NHS treatments 3
   sick days 3
economic pressures 2–5
employment standards 30
endocrine disorders 13
energy dense convenience foods 12
energy requirements 107
engaging participants 84
equipment in the workplace 1–2, 26

ergonomic factors 1–2, 25–7
ethnicity, and obesity 8–10
evacuation procedures 94–5
exercise recommendations 45–6
   see also physical activities

F-plan diet 110
families, patterns of obesity 12
fast foods 12
fat measurements 10
fat requirements 107
Ferrie, JE *et al.* 27–8
financial resources
   large budget options 64–6
   low budget options 61–4
   no budget options 58–61
Firmafrugt (Denmark) 72
fitness to work 23–5
   aerobic capacity 25
   physical agility 25
   work standards and criteria 33
food labelling 42–3, 58, 107–8
Food Standards Agency (FSA) 43
food substitutes 117
fruit and vegetables
   portion advice 42
   workplace initiatives 72
Fruitions Limited 65
functional limitations 23–4
future trends in obesity 11

gall bladder disease 19
gallstones 18
gastric bypass surgery 49
gastroplasty 49
gender
   prevalence of obesity 11
   sick leave absences 27
   wage discrepancies 33
General Electric Company (GEC) 72
genetic predisposition 11–12
GI diet 111–12
glandular problems 13
GlaxoSmithKline (GSK) 63
gout 18
government policies 4–5
grapefruit diet 110

guidelines
    for physical activities 45–6
    see also government policies;
        information sources
gyms and health clubs 64–6, 73

'halo' effect 32
Ham, TS *et al.* 20
health clubs and gyms 64–6, 73
health promotion programmes *see*
    interventions in the workplace
healthcare, access problems 36–7
healthcare workers
    attitudes towards obesity 35
    interventions to improve fitness
        80–1
healthy food options 117
    see also nutrition and diet education
Heart of Birmingham (HOB) 61
Hertz, RP *et al.* 28
hip and knee replacements 36
hypertension 17, 19
hypoglycaemic drugs 13

implantable gastric stimulation
    techniques 50
Indian Airlines 38
individual-based workplace
    interventions 83–92
information sources 99–103
    books and articles 99–100
    practical help for employees 102–3
    websites 100–2
insulin 13
interventions in the workplace 53–67,
    75–82
    background 53–4
    considerations and reasons 54–6
    health and safety issues 55
    influencing factors 56–7
    initial preparations 56–7
    initiatives based on budget
        availability 58–67
    moral and ethical aspects 56
    motivation factors 88–9
    progress problems 88
    selling the concept 57–8

suggested eight week programme
    113–15
undertaking individual assessments
    85–8
use of individual-based approaches
    83–92
use of population-based approaches
    77–82

jaw wiring 49
job types and obesity 28–9
joint replacements 36

Kennedy, DB and Homant, RJ 33
kidney cancer 18
kidney disease 18
Knock Travel (Belfast) 60, 61

labelling foods 42–3, 58, 107–8
labour market changes 2–3
laparoscopic banding 49
Larsson, UE and Mattsson, E 20
lawyers 81–2
legal aspects 93–7
    antidiscrimination legislation 31,
        32–3, 93–7
    categorisation of 'disability' 93–4
legal cases, *Cook vs Rhode Island
    Department of Mental Health,
    Retardation and Hospitals* ruling 32–3
life expectancies 1
    see also mortality data
lifestyle factors 12–14
    and retirement 27–8
liposuction 105
losing weight
    impact of diets 106
    patterns 44–5
    progress problems 88
    recommended rates 105–6
'low-fat' products 108

management of obesity 41–50
    commercial weight loss programmes
        46
    medical interventions 46–8
    nutritional approaches 41–5

management of obesity (*continued*)
  physical activities 45–6
  surgery 48–50
Mayo Clinic 71
measurement of obesity 7–10
  BMI's 7–10
  body fat estimations 10
medical problems 15–20
  cancers 18
  cardiovascular disease 17
  diabetes 15–17
  psychological consequences 19–20
  respiratory disease 17–18
  other conditions 19
medications *see* drugs causing obesity
meetings, standing up 71
menorrhagia 18
menues 70–1
Merseyside Travelwise 63–4
Merthyr Tydfil Housing association 59
metabolic syndrome 8–10, 17
mobility problems 25
mortality data 15
  see also life expectancies
motivation factors 88–9
myocardial infarction 19

NHS treatments, economic costs 3
night eating syndrome 19–20
'no progress' 88
nutrition and diet education 41–5
  general guidelines 42
  healthy lunch options 117
  information sources 100–2
  labelling of food 42–3, 58, 107–8
  population-based strategies 80
  portion sizes 43–4
  restaurant/canteen changes 119
  workplace interventions 58–67
  workplace recommendations
    119–21

obese people
  and disability classifications 93–7
  employment experiences 38
  fitness problems 23–5
  health conditions 15–20

pay and promotion prospects 23,
  31–3
perceptions of public attitudes 34
obesity
  causes 11–14
  classifications 8
  definitions 7–8
  economic costs 3
  extent of the problem 1–2, 11
  measurement 7–10
  prevalence 1, 11
  projections 11
obesogenic drugs *see* drugs causing
  obesity
occupations types and weight gain
  28–9
oesophageal cancer 18
office equipment 1–2
office jobs, workplace interventions
  78–80
oral contraceptives 13
organisation and design initiatives
  69–73
Orlistat 47
osteoarthritis 19
ovarian cancer 19

parents, patterns of obesity 12
patient groups 102–3
pay 31–2
pedometers 59–60, 63, 71
personal protective equipment (PPE)
  26–7, 55
physical activities
  guidelines 45–6
  individual-based programmes 90–1
  information sources 101, 102
  population-based strategies 78–82
  reduced levels and obesity 12
  workplace initiatives 59–67
  workplace recommendations
    121–2
physical agility 25
physical consequences of obesity *see*
  medical problems
Pitney Bowes (US) 76–7
polycystic ovary syndrome (PCOS) 18

population-based interventions 77–82
portion sizes 12, 43–4
prejudice and discrimination issues 2, 31–8
   attitudes and challenges 31–5
   impact on healthcare access 36–7
   personal accounts 38
   public and customer responses 37
prevalence of obesity 1, 11
Prochaska, JO and DiClemente, CC 89
programmes *see* interventions in the workplace
progress problems 88
promotion prospects 23
   see also salaries and wages
protective overclothes and aprons 26, 55
protein requirements 108
psychological wellbeing, public perceptions 33–4

Radisson SAS Hotel (Edinburgh) 70–1
recruiting individuals 85
research studies, impact of physical appearances 31–2
respiratory disease 17–18
respiratory equipment 27
restaurant/canteen meals 12, 119
retirement 27–8
Rimonabant 48
Roe, DA and Eickwort, KR 33
Roehling, M 33
Rosemary Conley's hip and thigh diet 110

safety issues 55
St George's University (West Indies) 60
salaries and wages 31–3
sales executives 81–2
salt intake 105, 108
sandwich vendors 120
Saport, I and Halpern, JJ 31–2
Selecta 74
Sibutramine 47
sick absences 3, 23, 27–8
sleep apnoea 17–18

Slimfast meals 110
smoking cessation 13
snoring 17–18
South Beach diet 111
stab vests 26
standards and criteria for jobs 33
stereotypes 33, 34
subsidised meals 71–2
sugar 107
'super sizing' 12
support groups 102–3
surgery 48–50

Telus (Canada) 65
treadmill use 71
truck drivers 82
truncal obesity *see* abdominal fat

uniforms 23, 27
United Kingdom
   future trends 11
   prevalence of obesity 1, 11
United States
   ACOEM Labor Day Checklist 123–5
   antidiscrimination legislation 32–3
   future trends 11
   prevalence of obesity 11
uterine cancer 18

varicose veins 18
vending machines 74
   healthy options 119–20
vertical banded gastroplasty 49

walking 45
   within work situations 79–80, 81
water dispensers 79, 80
websites 100–2
weight loss programmes (commercial) 46
weight reduction *see* interventions in the workplace; losing weight
Weight Watchers programmes 109
Whitehall study (Ferrie *et al.*) 27–8
Williams, NR and Malik, N 24

work ability 23–45
Work Fit initiative (BT) 90–1
workplaces
    environmental and equipment issues
      1–2, 26–7, 94–5
    functional impact of obese
      employees 23–4
    health improvement opportunities
      53–67
    health promotion programmes
      75–82

    layouts and ergonomic factors 1–2,
      26–7, 79, 94–5
    organisation and work design
      initiatives 69–73
    use of individual-based interventions
      83–92
    use of population-based
      interventions 77–82
workstations 26

Zone diet 111